Medicine is the Best Laughter

A Second Dose

Medicine is the Best Laughter

A Second Dose

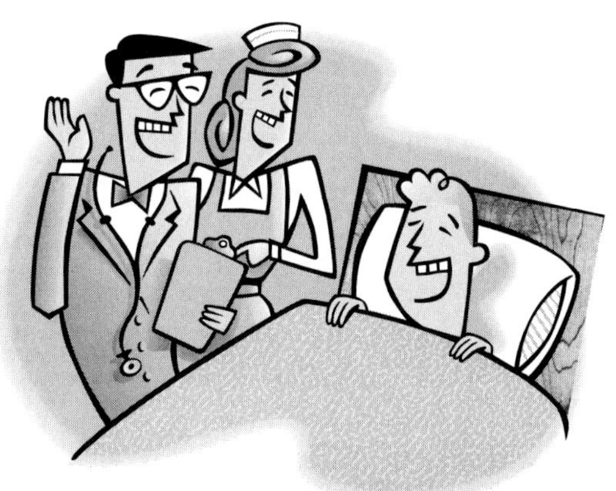

Mosby

St. Louis Baltimore Boston Carlsbad Chicago Minneapolis New York Philadelphia Portland
London Milan Sydney Tokyo Toronto

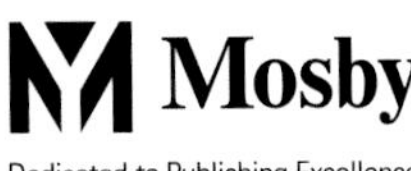

Dedicated to Publishing Excellence

A Times Mirror
Company

Publisher: Anne S. Patterson
Editor: Susie H. Baxter
Developmental Editor: Ellen Baker Geisel
Project Manager: Gayle May Morris
Manufacturing Manager: Don Carlisle
Design and Cover Illustration: Reed Darmon

Printed in the United States of America
Printing/binding by R.R. Donnelley
Cover printing by Pinnacle Press, Inc

Mosby, Inc.
11830 Westline Industrial Drive
St. Louis, Missouri 63146

International Standard Book Number 0-8151-9640-7

98 99 00 01 02 / 9 8 7 6 5 4 3 2 1

To my mother
Dorka Bosker, who
makes me laugh
with the best of them

Preface

Medical humor is alive and well. Since publication of the first edition of *Medicine Is The Best Laughter*, I have continued my systematic search for cartoons that would make a beeline to the funny bone of both medical professionals and the lay public. Fortunately, piles and piles of gut-splitting, marrow-tickling material has found its way to my mailbox, fax machine, and e-mail over the past three years. This "Second Dose" of *Medicine Is The Best Laughter* is the result of my continuing hunt for the ultimate medical cartoons.

In fact, because the first edition reached such a wide and diverse audience, I have become somewhat of a magnet for physicians, nurses, and other health professionals who have been kind enough to share their favorite gags and cartoons with me. During the course of my travels across America, lecturing at medical schools and hospitals about drug prescribing in "chronologically gifted" individuals, I have often been approached by an audience member—usually a physician, nurse, or pharmacist—clutching a stack of photocopied cartoons. In a flash, cartoons are whizzing before my eyes, and my new-found friend is suggesting something like, "Dr. Bosker, I think these would be a hoot for the next edition of your book. Do you think you can use any of them?"

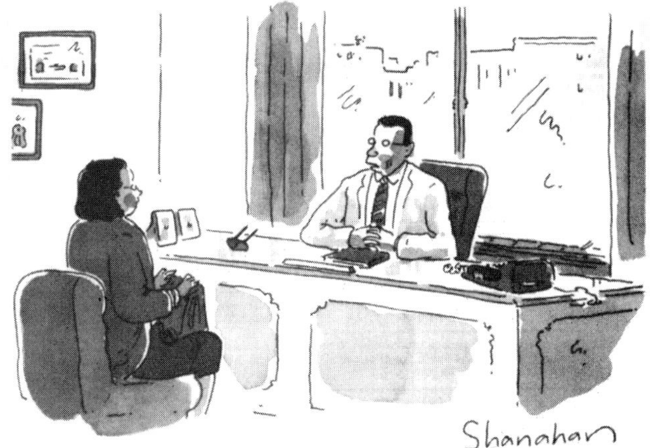

"You can rest assured, Mrs. Wilson, that your husband will receive the best care known to medical coverage."

As you might expect, many of these curbside offerings from humor enthusiasts have made their way into the current volume. And for good reason. Medical humor afficionados that I know are an obsessed and devoted bunch who comb daily papers and magazines—and increasingly, the Internet—in search of knee-slapping, teeth-flashing gems that look at the lighter side of what is a very serious profession.

In particular, I remember the twinkle-eyed pathologist from Miami who pointed me to the *New Yorker* cartoon in which an attending physician says to his patient, "Congratulations, you have made the most remarkable recovery from an autopsy I have ever seen. "And, of course, I will never forget the Chicago psychiatrist, whose therapy suite was draped with more than 50 framed medical cartoons. He recommended the Sydney Harris cartoon in which a couple is setting their table for a dinner party, and the host advises his wife: "Let's seat the guests like this—a manic, then a depressive; a manic, then a depressive . . . . "An endocrinologist from Atlanta was absolutely certain that I would want to include the cartoon in which a physician counsels his overweight patient: "It's partly glandular and partly 8500 calories per day," or the companion piece in which the doctor explains, "The problem is, you're retaining ice cream." He was right. I have included them in this collection without hesistation.

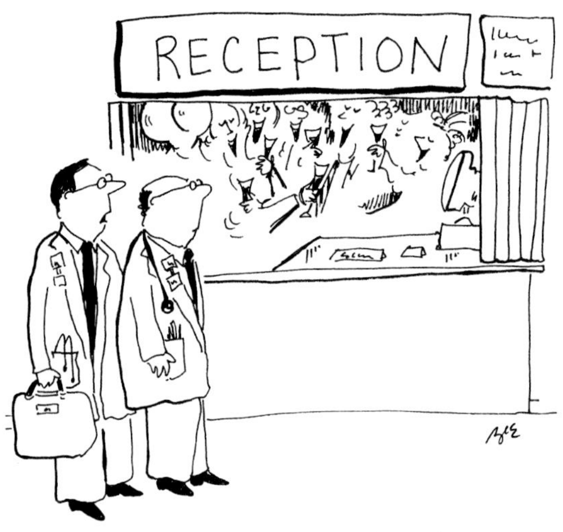

"We better change that sign."

Some physicians insist that in the high-tech, neuron-probing world of modern medicine, the window to the soul is the PET scan, the human genome, or the mini-mental status examination. They may have a point, but I have come to believe that, in the real day-to-day world, the true window of the soul is the break room refrigerator or the glass partition panel in the clinic waiting room, on which nurses, physicians, and other health care providers affix their favorite examples of medical humor.

Check out a physician's, pharmacist's, or nurse's bookshelf and you'll know what their intellectual interests are and what area of medicine they specialize in; but check out the cartoons that are slathered on their refrigerator or bulletin board, and you'll make a beeline to the interstices of his or her soul. With cartoons as a looking glass, you'll instantly know how someone sees themself, what predicaments of current medical practice they consider of the highest priority, and, most importantly, how they view the world.

The family practitioner who posts a cartoon in his medication sample closet in which an office receptionist advises a departing patient, "And don't forget to take some of our complimentary antibiotics on the way out," tells you what her attitude might be toward the pharmaceutical industry. Similarly, a psychiatrist who has a poster-size Gary Larsen cartoon in which a therapist jots the words, "Just plain nuts!" on his notepad might be broadcasting early symptoms of burnout. The gynecologist who has taped a cartoon on her office desk lamp in which one woman confides to another, "That's right Eleanor, I divorced Harry and replaced him with estrogen!" is certainly showing us how she views the never-ending struggle between romance and personal pharmacology, especially as it relates to hormone replacement therapy. Finally, the geriatrician who has taped up a cartoon, in which one of two senior citizens playing poker says to the other, "I'll see your two Valium and raise you three Zoloft," is making a statement about the pitfalls of polypharmacy in the elderly.

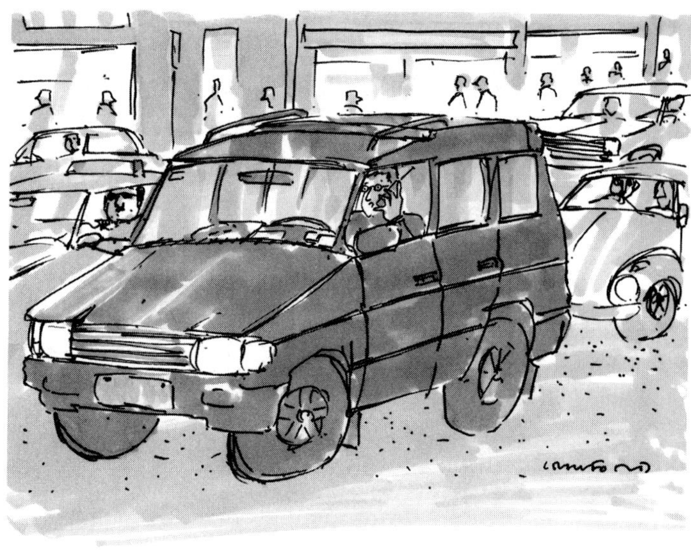

"You think I would have sunk forty thousand clams into this lemon if I had known they were coming out with a nine-dollar boner pill?"

Although medical cartoons may be seen by thousands of people, the beauty of being on the receiving end of one is that viewing a cartoon is a very personal experience that frequently becomes a long-running private joke. Even after the newsprint may have yellowed from too much sunlight, and long after a cartoon may have been smudged with a coffee stain, or ripped by a reckless elbow or fingernail, it often continues as a beacon of pleasure for its owner, tickling our laugh centers day after day, even after multiple viewings.

Some of the cartoons in this category—i.e., those that have stood the test of time and continue to grow on me—include the one in which a man with multiple gunshot wounds to his chest is sitting on the examination table and the physician says: "Those bullet holes are something new, aren't they?" And I still get a kick out of the cartoon in which a physician suggests that, "Before we try assisted suicide, I think we should give aspirin a chance." Finally, there is the nativity scene in which the Virgin Mary, holding the baby Jesus on her lap, is informed that she'll have to go home because her "insurance doesn't cover more than one day in the manger."

Perhaps even more than editorials, commentaries, or op-ed pieces, medical cartoons have a way of cutting to the quick and splaying open the essence of political, scientific, or social issues that impinge on the world of health care. What better way to express the dramatic impact of a new "potency pill" than with a cartoon in which a man driving a Land Rover speaks to his friend on a cell phone and complains: "You think I would have spent 40,000 clams on this lemon if I'd known they were coming out with a nine dollar boner pill!" The fierce debate surrounding quality cutbacks in HMOs and other capitated health plans is summarized in a cartoon in which an insurance adjuster apologetically informs the patient that, "I'm sorry, but our health plan does not cover pre-exisiting organs."

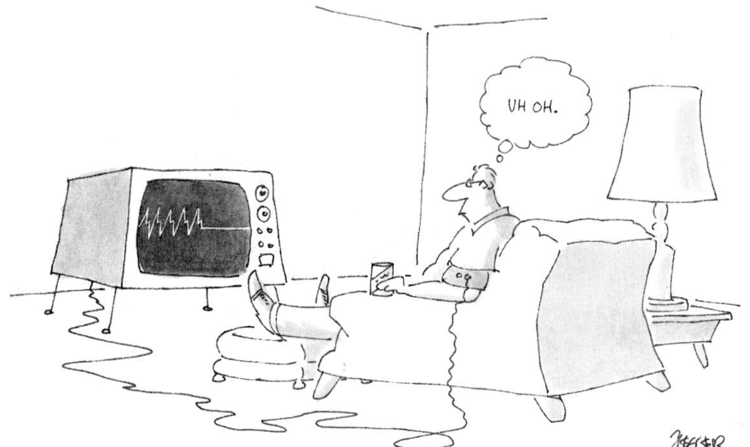

More than ever before, medically oriented cartoons have entered the comic mainstream and have pushed the edge of humor, in general, to new limits. It's about time. In the 1930s and 1940s, the cartoonist occupied a place in the cultural hierarchy not far below the movie star or inventor. And even writers with the stature of John Updike have applied themselves to deciphering the magic of cartoons, and recognized that "cartoons have personalities whose recognition the informed mind attains before any conscious sorting out of traits, just as we spot a known face, or even a certain swing of the body, at a distance that blurs all details."

Judging from at least one cartoon that I have taped to my office wall, I am not the only person who recognizes the impact that medical humor has on the human psyche, and perhaps, even on physical well-being. In this cartoon, a pharmaceutical company CEO stands at a dais in front of his stock shareholders and warns: "Our research shows that laughter, not medications, are the best medicine."

Gideon Bosker, MD
May, 1998

Acknowledgments

This book required the collaboration and cooperation of many individuals and institutions. First and foremost, I would like to thank the principal actors in the drama—the cartoonists, artists, and humorists whose work has graced the pages of America's finest publications and found its way into the various libraries, archives, and collections throughout the country. In this regard, I owe a special debts to Bob Mankoff, *New Yorker* cartoonist- and archivist par excellence, who did everything in his power to ensure that I would have the finest and funniest cartoons for inclusion in this edition.

I would especially like to thank Mittie Hellmich, who provided expert editorial, research, and illustrational skills throughout the project. I am especially indebted to Reed Darmon, the book's designer and cover illustrator, who conceived an elegant cover design, and ensured that the cartoons were presented in a manner that ensured this book would be a visual feast.

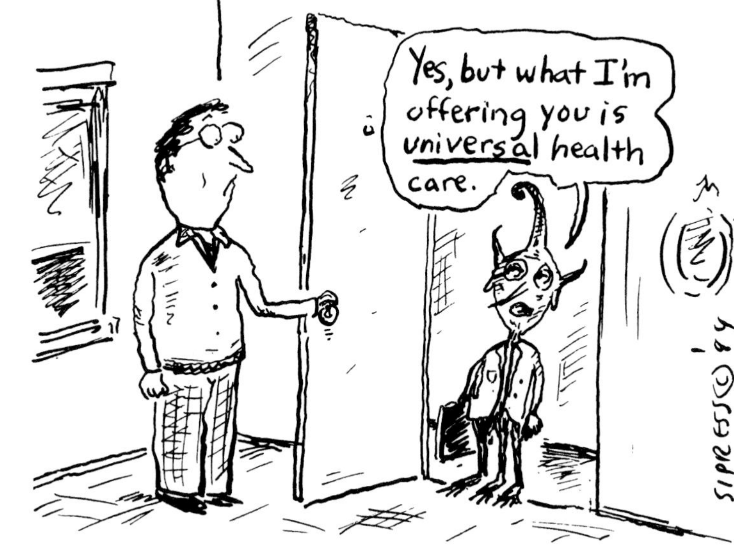

I sincerely appreciate the support of the Mosby editorial team, which has demonstrated its deep commitment to the project, beginning with the first edition, and once again provided wise counsel in the area of book design, implementation, and cartoon selection. I owe special thanks to Colleen Boyd, whose organizational skills were key to the development of the book.

For her encourgement, strategic thinking, and creative planning, I would like to thank my editor, Susie Baxter, who laid the groundwork for a book that would reach a much wider audience—both professional and non-professional. Her wise counsel was appreciated at every stage of the project and this edition of the book reflects her editorial panache and publishing savvy.

I especially am grateful to Ellen Baker Geisel, my develomental editor, who offered many hours at various stages of the project and whose suggestions for refinements and fine-tuning were always on the mark. If anyone can be credited for cajoling and humoring me to see this project through to its completion, it is Ellen, who supplied me with the world's funniest cartoons, FAXes, and e-mails. They not only kept me laughing, but suggested novel and more humorous directions this edition might take.

Finally, there are all my friends, colleagues, and family members who took the time to clip cartoons, tell me jokes over long distance phone lines, and who spent countless hours poring over hundreds of cartoons in order to identify the funniest in the bunch. In this regard, I would like to thank Joanne Day, David Wilson, Bianca Lencek-Bosker, Lena Lencek, Dorothy Bosker, Hollis Wilde, Gene MacDonald, Margaret Mays, Richard Pine, and scores of other humor-loving people from around the world.

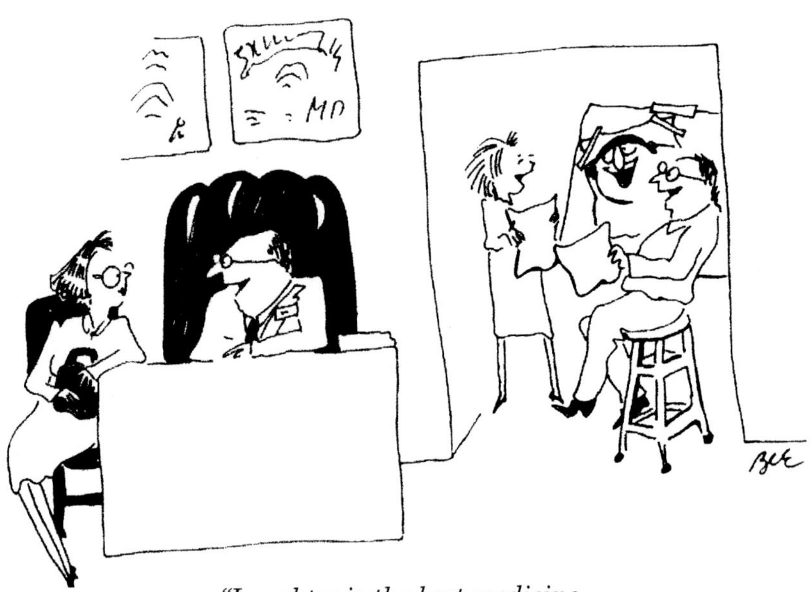

*"Laughter is the best medicine.
Please see the cartoonist on your way out."*

C O N T E N T S

Medicine is the Best Laughter

A Second Dose

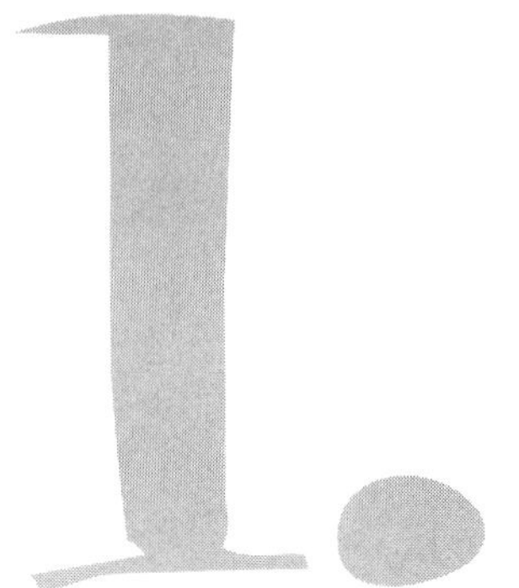

Badside Manners

Pronouncements at the bedside

Strange and unusual approaches to patient care

Patient-physician interactions

Dingy diagnoses

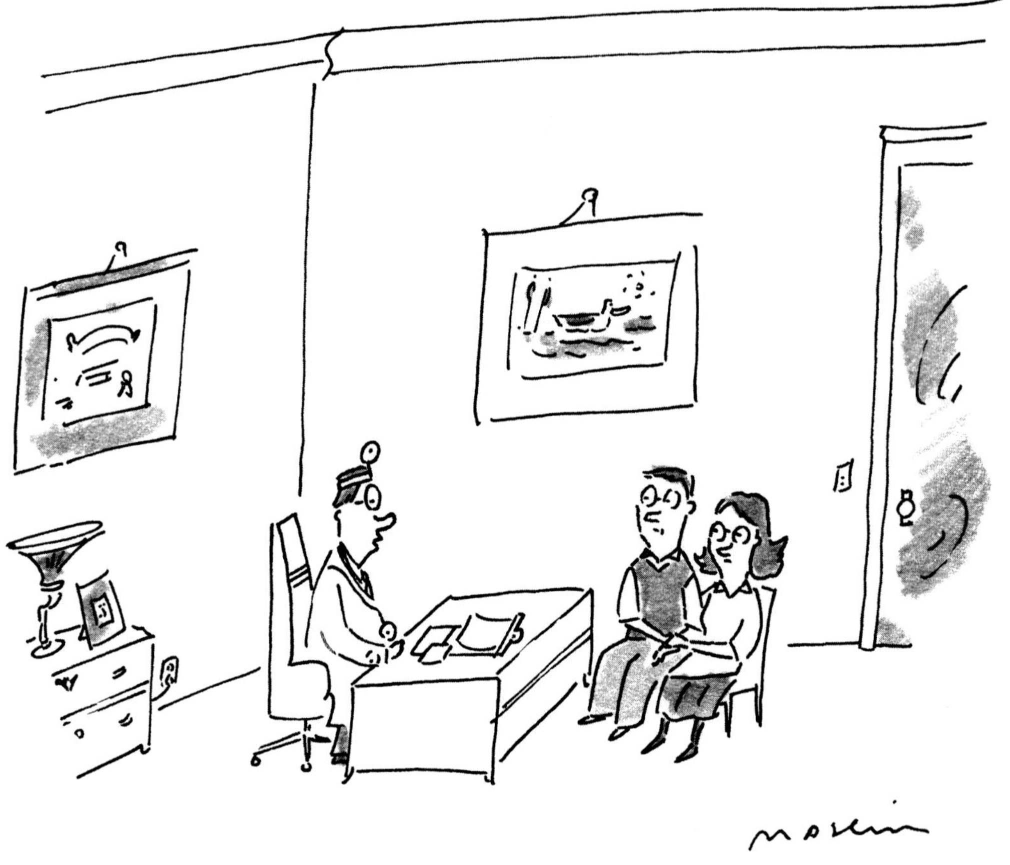

"No, I haven't performed the procedure myself, but I've seen it done successfully on 'E.R.' and 'Chicago Hope.'"

MISTER BOFFO by Joe Martin

A TIME TO WORRY
I'LL BE HONEST WITH YOU...
WHAT YOU HAVE IS SO RARE WE'RE NOT EVEN SURE THAT WE'RE PRONOUNCING IT RIGHT.

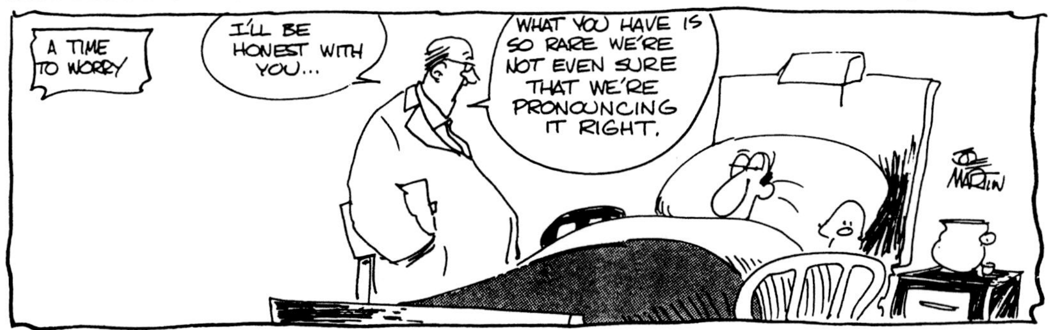

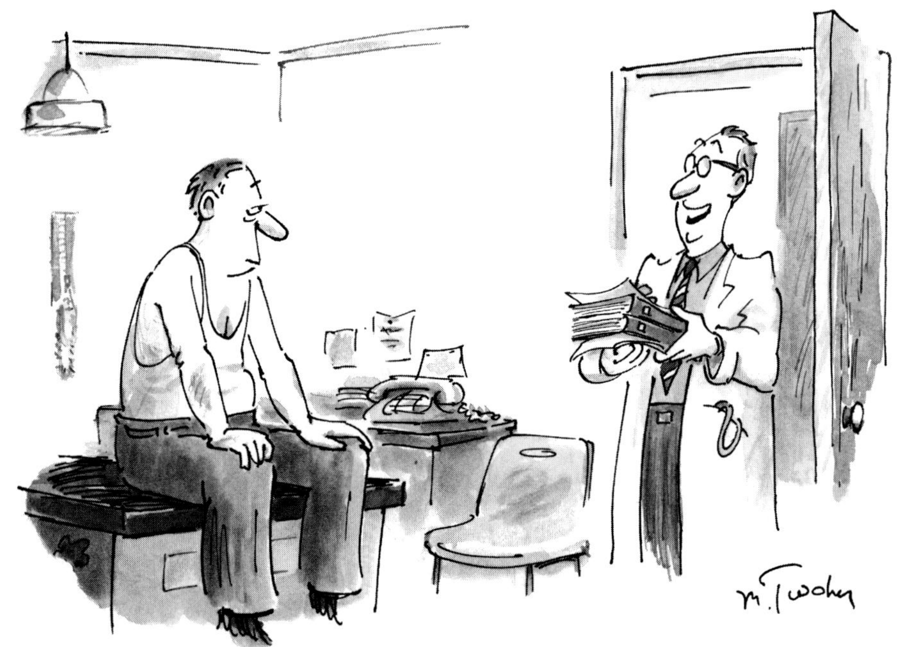

"Ah, Mr. Bromley. Nice to put a face on a disease."

HERMAN®

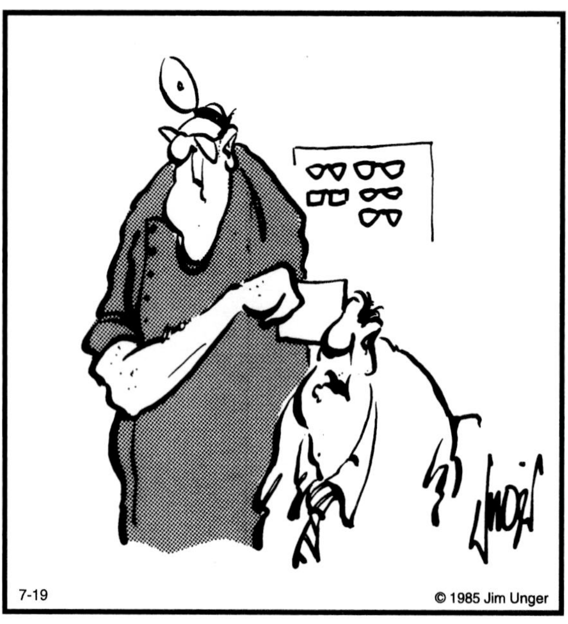

"I don't think I can read the card. You're holding it too close."

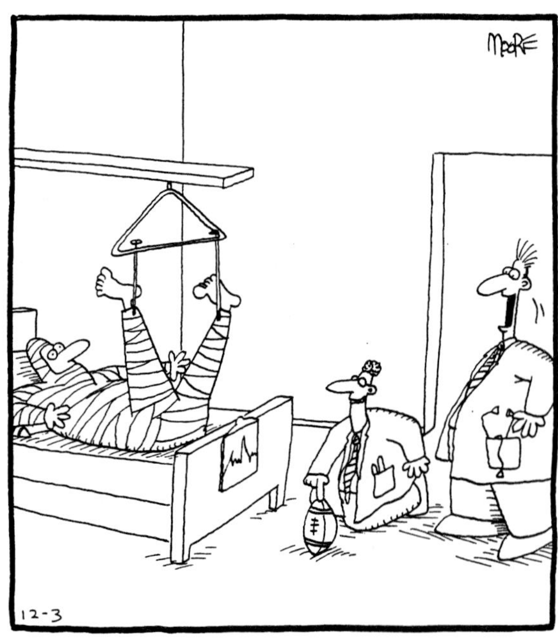

"OK, my turn...Cinderella story. Super Bowl is tied in overtime. Two seconds left. A field goal can win it all..."

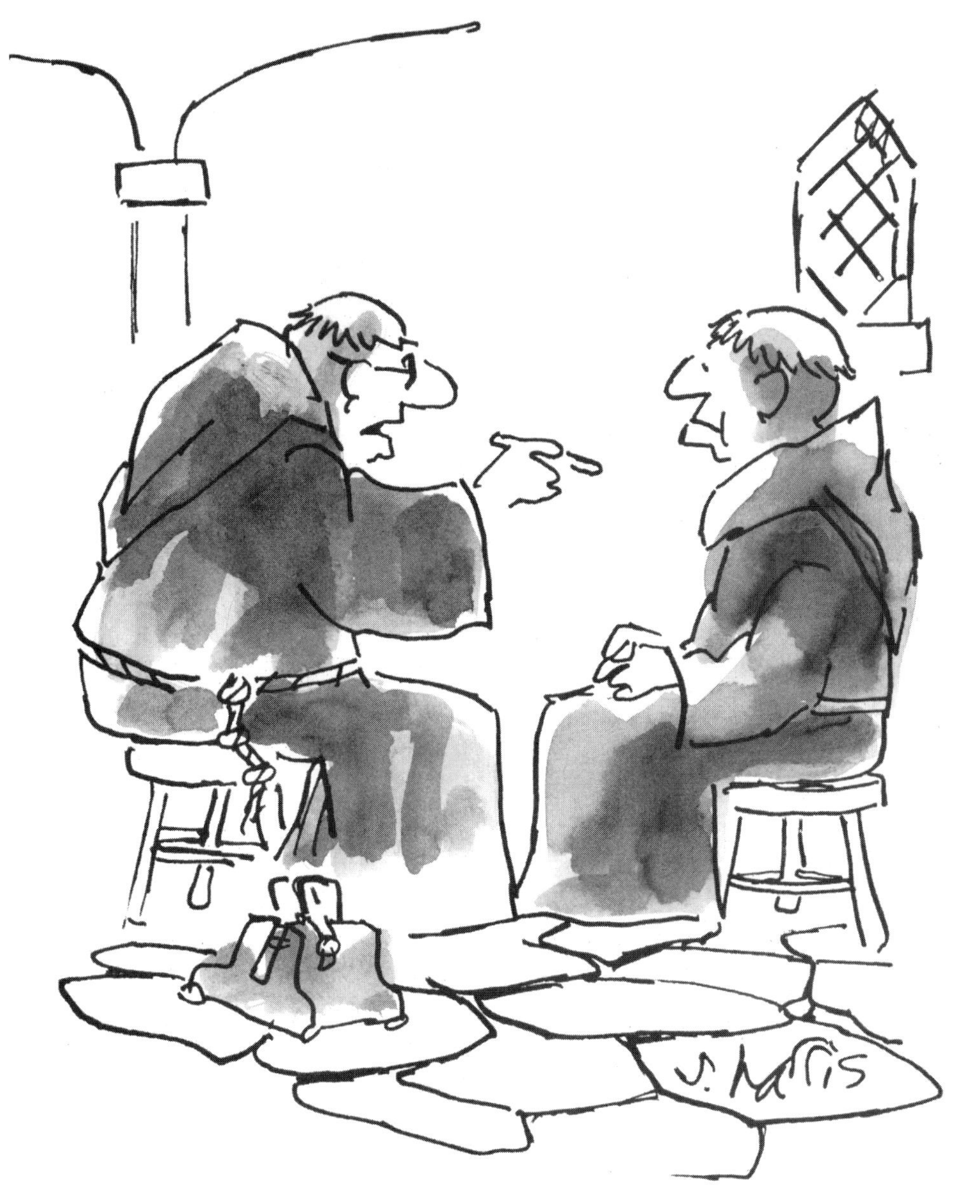

"Never mind your vow of silence — say 'Ah'."

HERMAN®

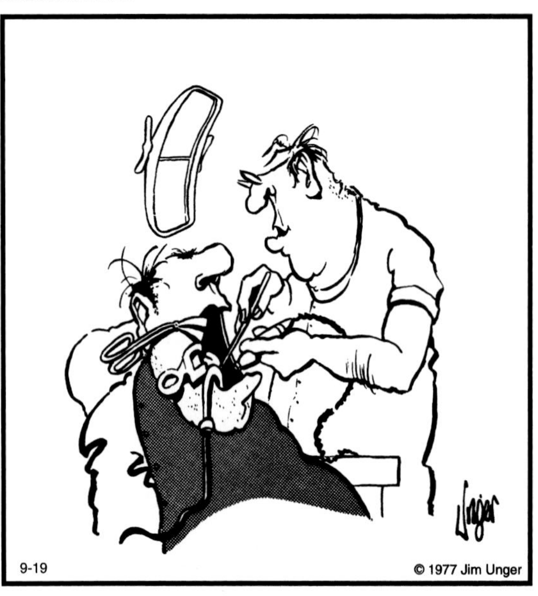

"Do you think the current economic policies will do anything to ease the unemployment problem?"

GOOD MORNING, AND WELCOME TO DR. BINGSLEY'S WAITING ROOM! TODAY'S FEATURED PRESENTATION WILL BE GANDHI, FOLLOWED BY DR. ZHIVAGO AT 2:00 P.M.
McPHERSON
7-3

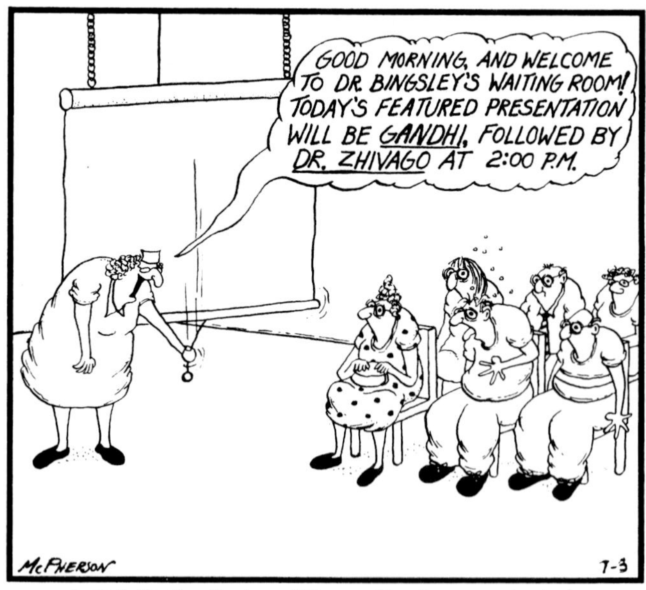

A definite sign that you'll be waiting for your doctor's appointment much longer than expected.

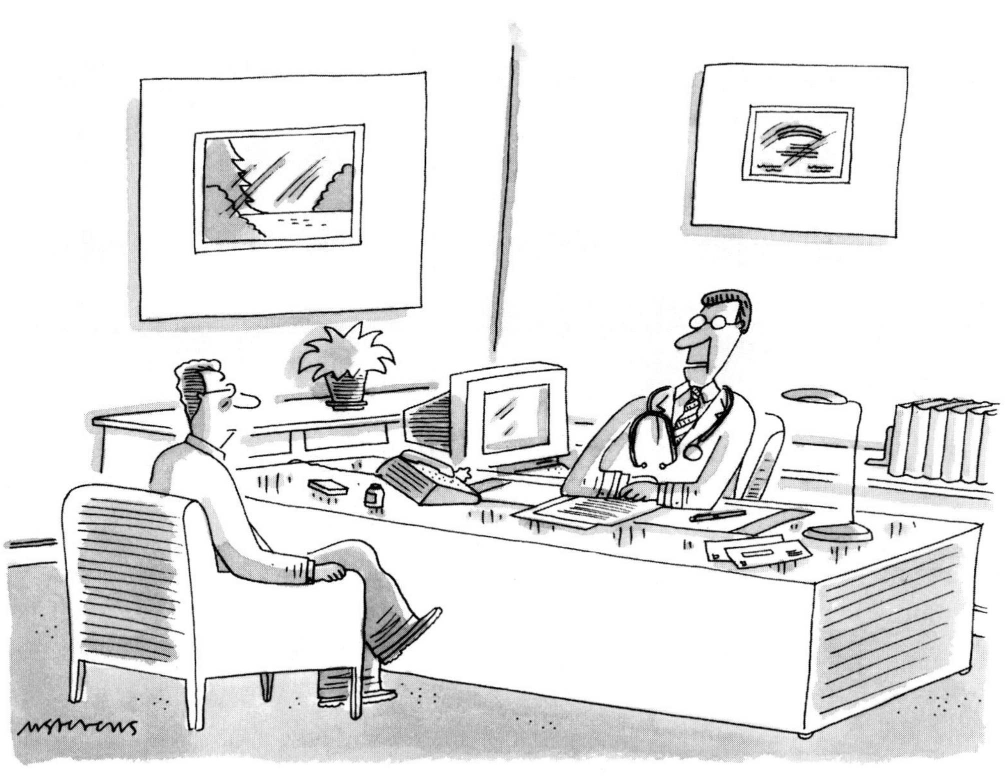

"Your condition is serious, Mr. Reynolds, but fortunately I recently scored some excellent weed that should alleviate your symptoms."

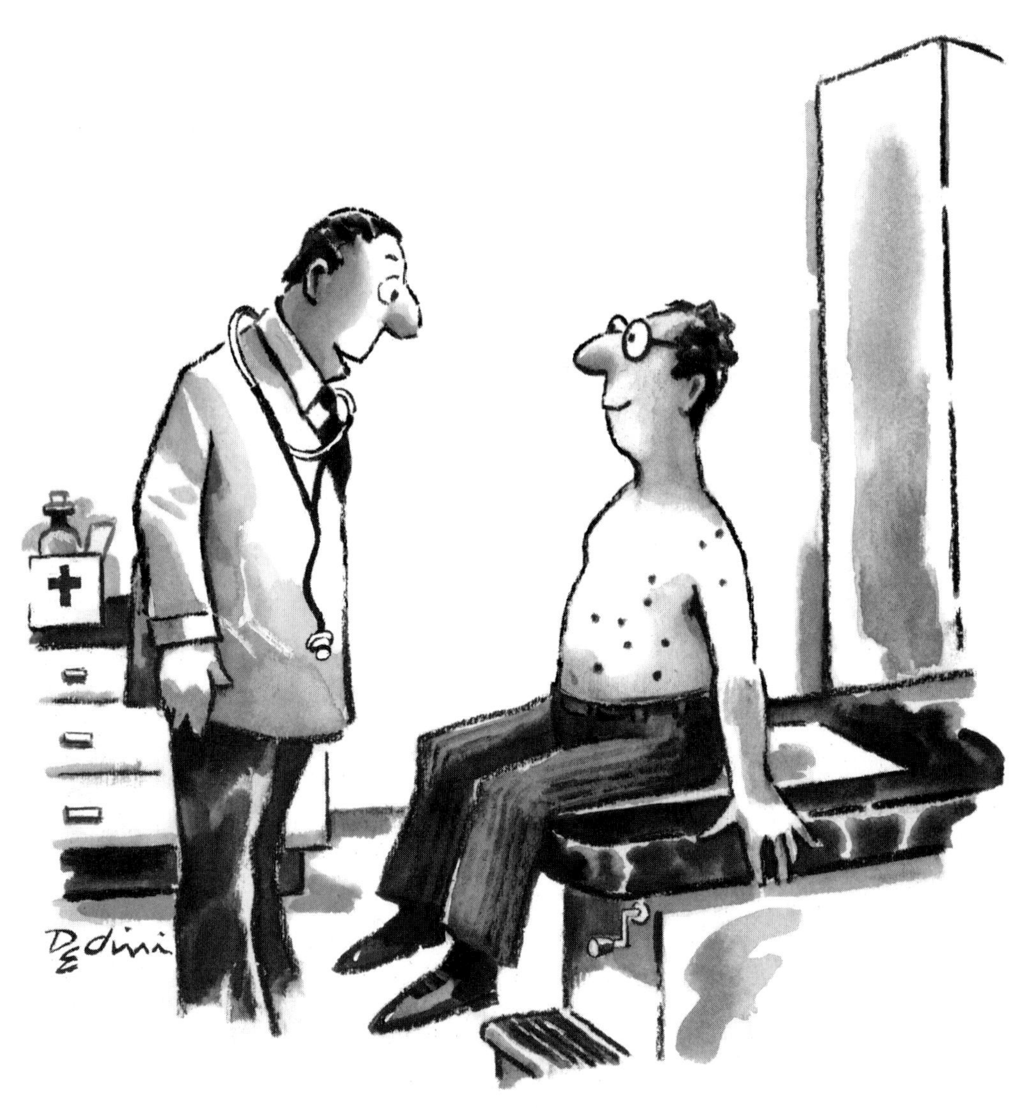

"Those bullet holes are something new, aren't they?"

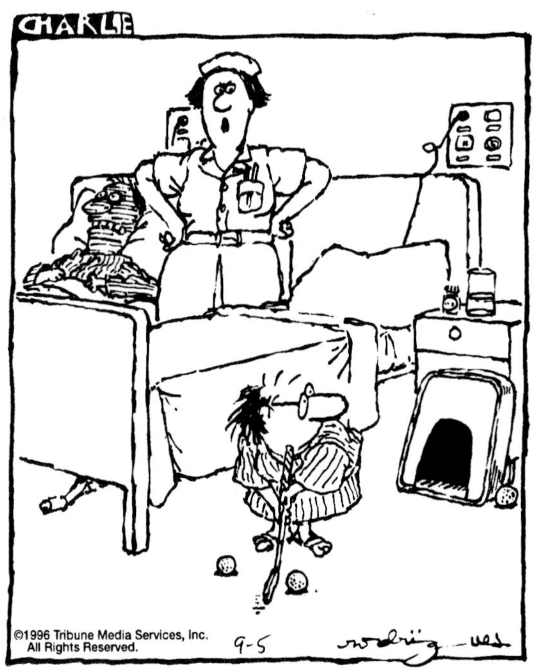

"Charr-lie, Mr. Spagnoli is waiting!"

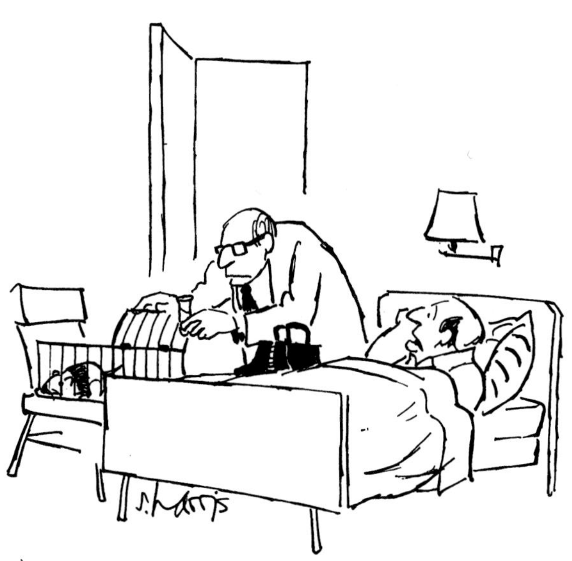

"You mean you're going to test it on a guinea pig now?*"*

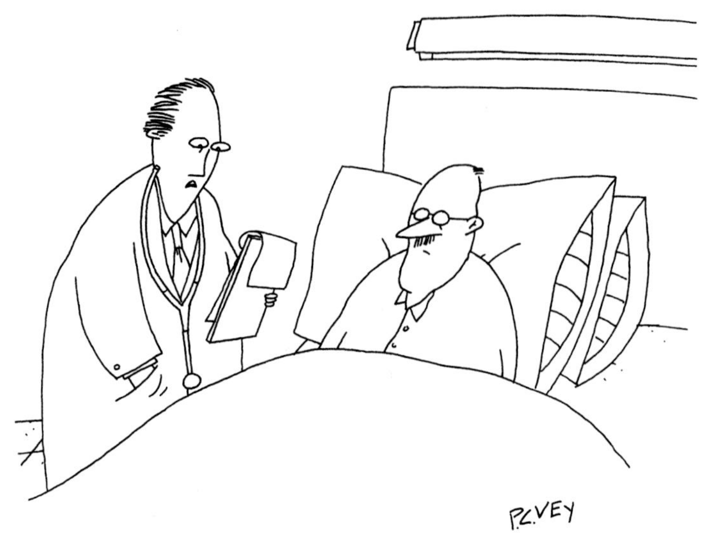

"As far as we can tell, Mr. Schroeder, your glasses are smudged."

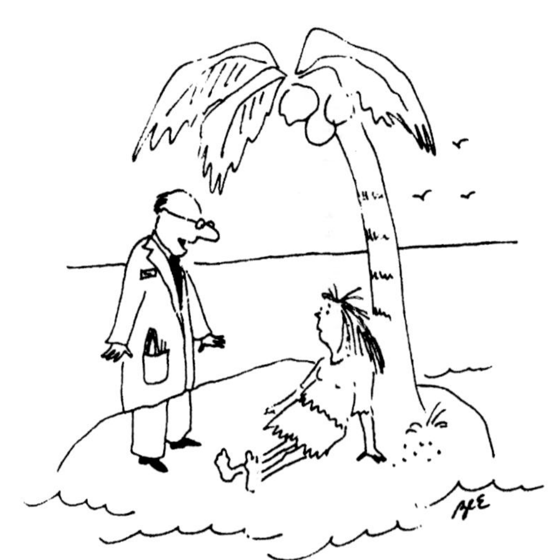

"Of course, feel free to get a second opinion."

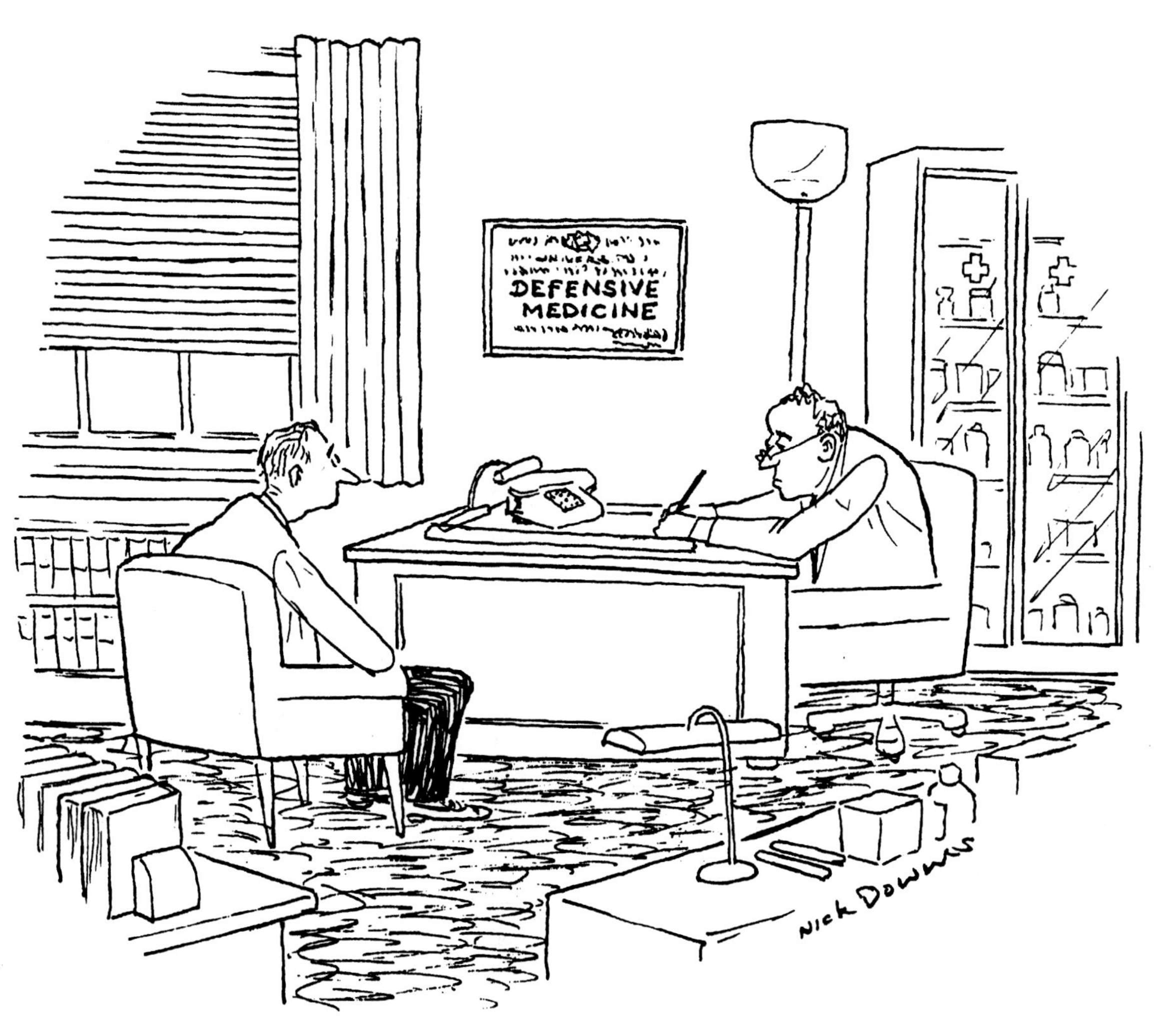
DEFENSIVE
MEDICINE
NICK DOWNES

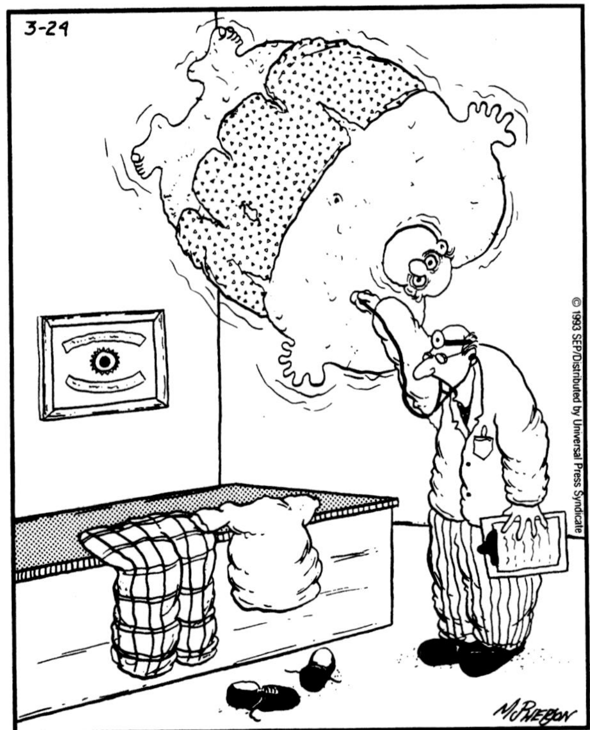

"Exhale."

UH...F? I MEAN H?!... NO WAIT... FOR CRYIN' OUT LOUD! I'M GONNA NEED THE HUBBLE TELESCOPE TO CORRECT MY EYESIGHT!
McPHERSON

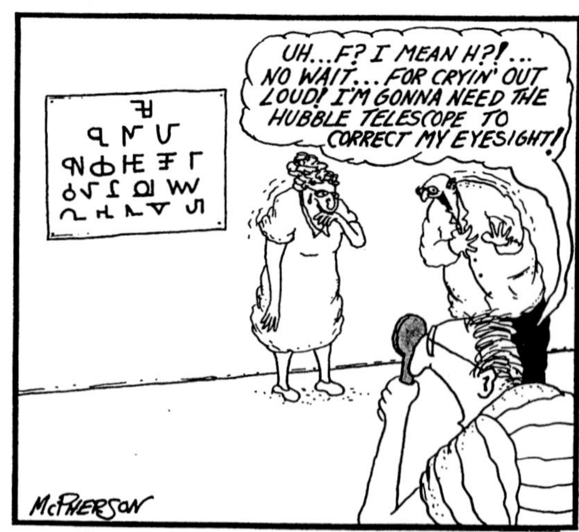

Every now and then, Dr. Walston liked to put up his joke eye chart.

Calvin and Hobbes

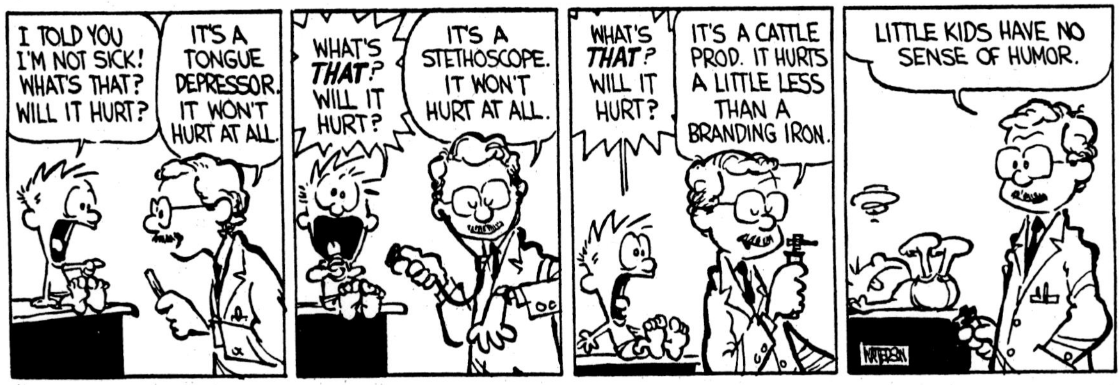

I TOLD YOU I'M NOT SICK! WHAT'S THAT? WILL IT HURT?
IT'S A TONGUE DEPRESSOR. IT WON'T HURT AT ALL.
WHAT'S *THAT*? WILL IT HURT?
IT'S A STETHOSCOPE. IT WON'T HURT AT ALL.
WHAT'S *THAT*? WILL IT HURT?
IT'S A CATTLE PROD. IT HURTS A LITTLE LESS THAN A BRANDING IRON.
LITTLE KIDS HAVE NO SENSE OF HUMOR.

HERMAN®

A
B C
5-15
© 1987 Jim Unger

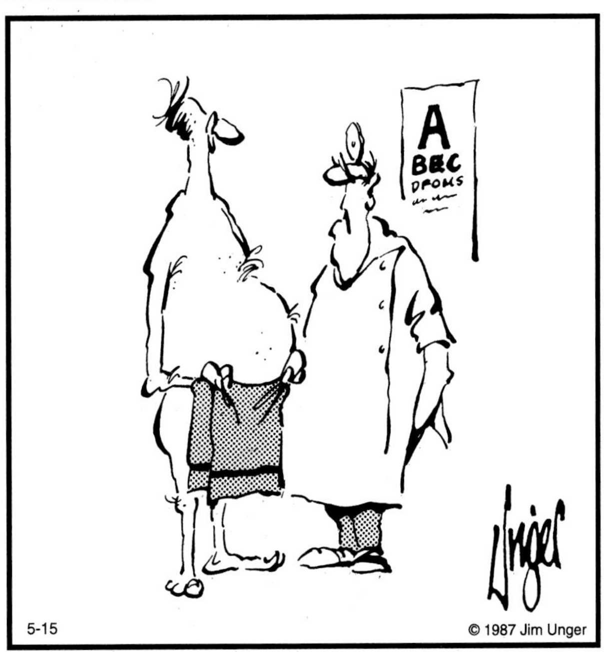

"Is this the first time you've had your eyes tested?"

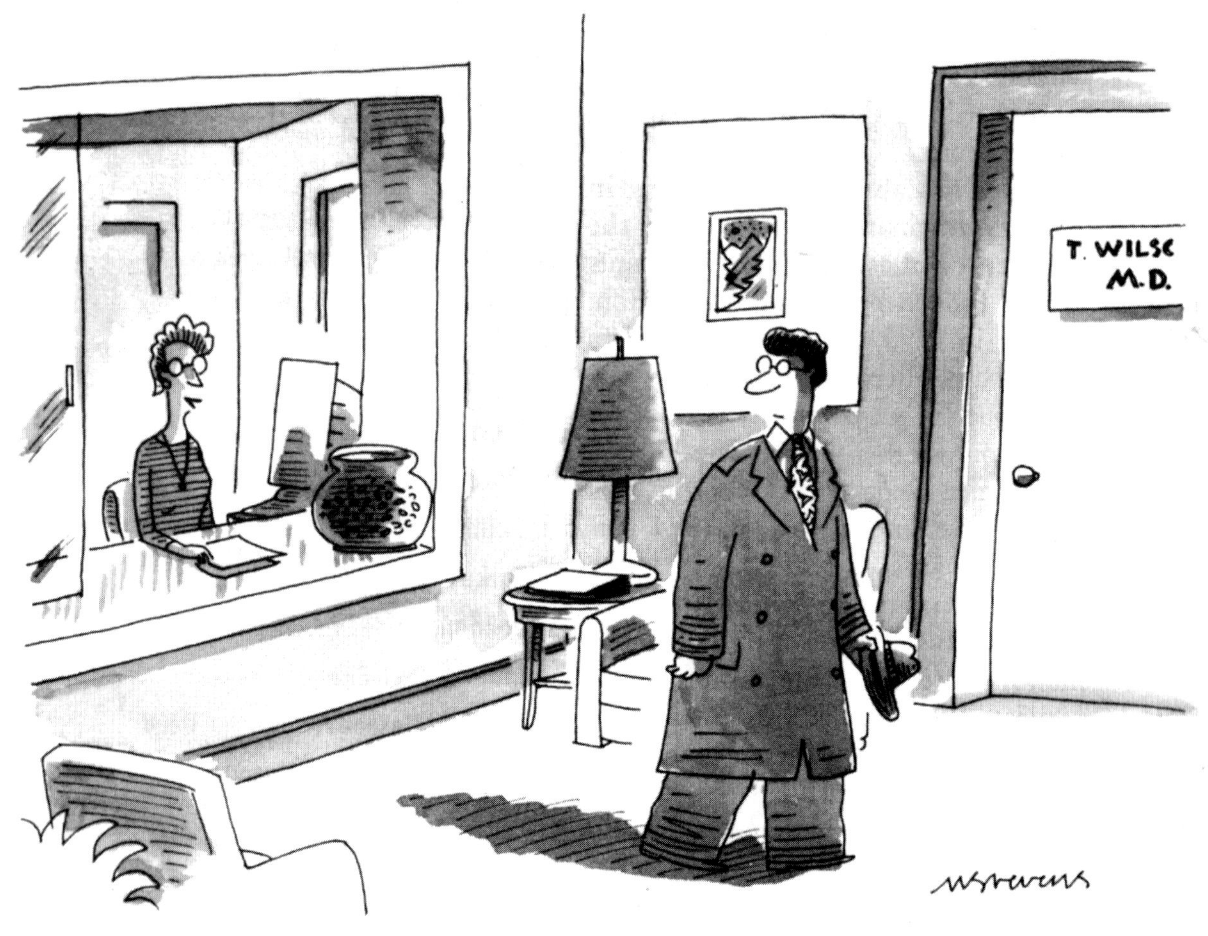

"Don't forget to take a handful of our complimentary antibiotics on your way out."

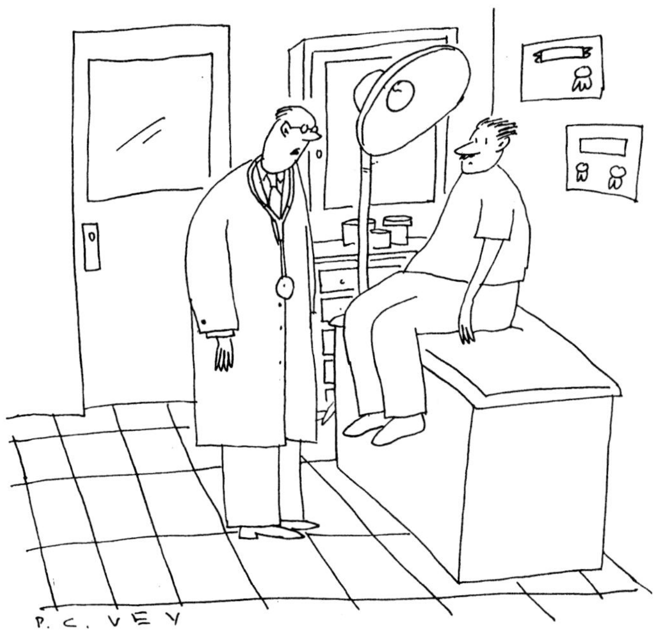

"This may be just because I'm a Doctor, but I would like to examine you."

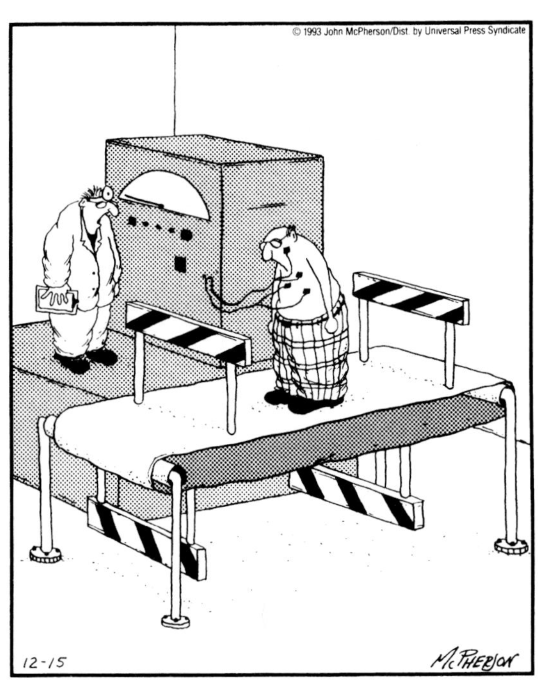

"You'll probably find this considerably more strenuous than other treadmill tests you've taken."

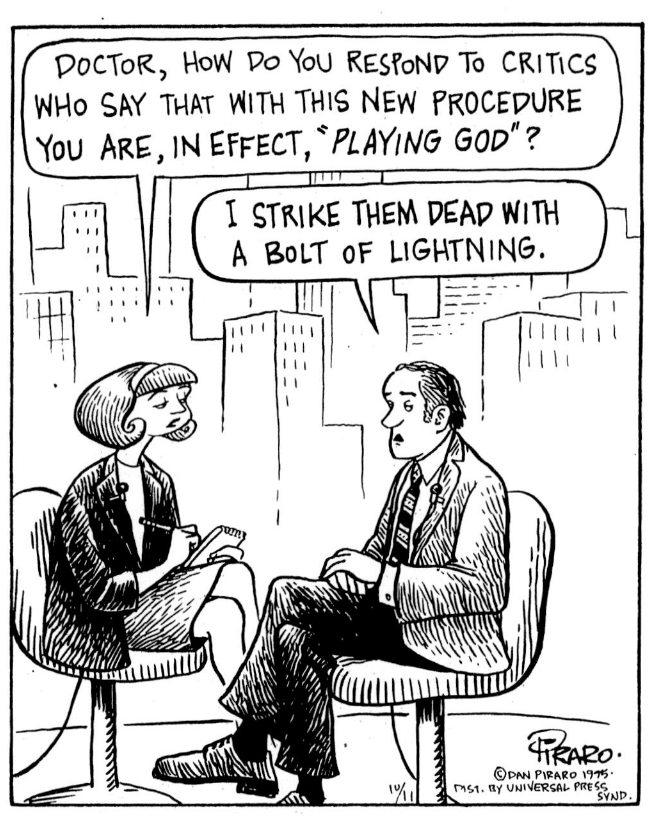
DOCTOR, HOW DO YOU RESPOND TO CRITICS WHO SAY THAT WITH THIS NEW PROCEDURE YOU ARE, IN EFFECT, "PLAYING GOD"?
I STRIKE THEM DEAD WITH A BOLT OF LIGHTNING.
PIRARO.
©DAN PIRARO 1995. DIST. BY UNIVERSAL PRESS SYND.

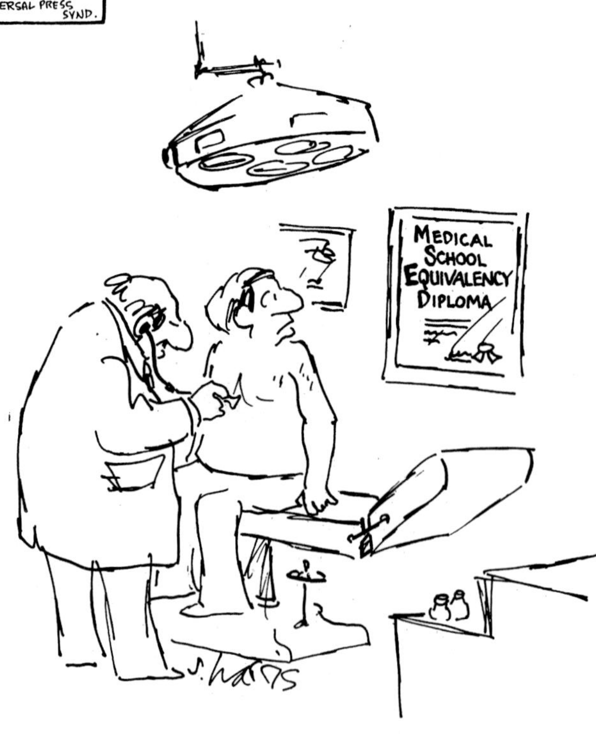
MEDICAL SCHOOL EQUIVALENCY DIPLOMA

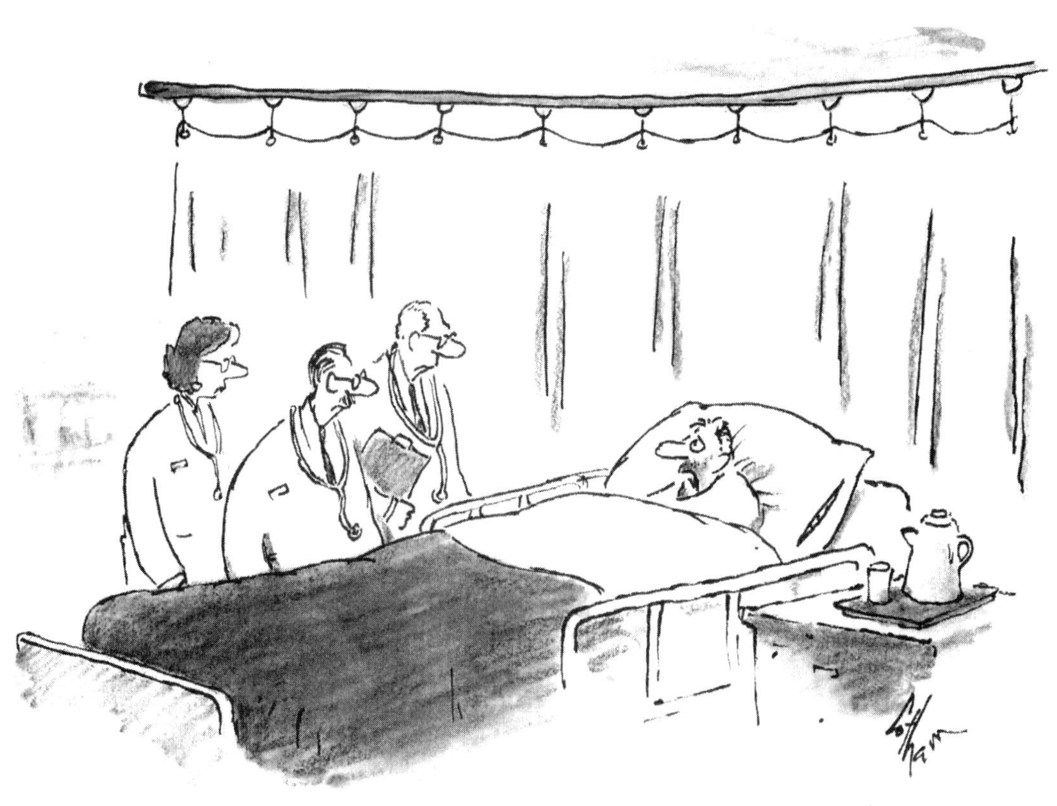

"But at the press conference you said I was going to be okay."

K.V.HACKLEY
M.D.
S. Harris

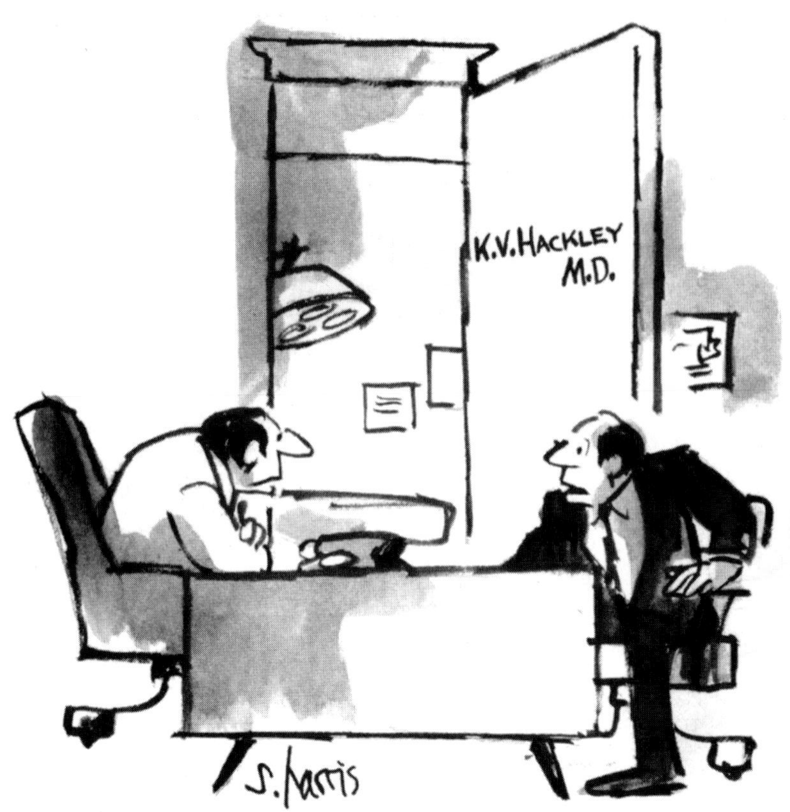

" 'Hackley's Syndrome'? But Dr. Grottmark said it was 'Grottmark's Syndrome.' "

YOU'RE GONNA FEEL A LITTLE STICK.
EARLY BLOOD DRAW

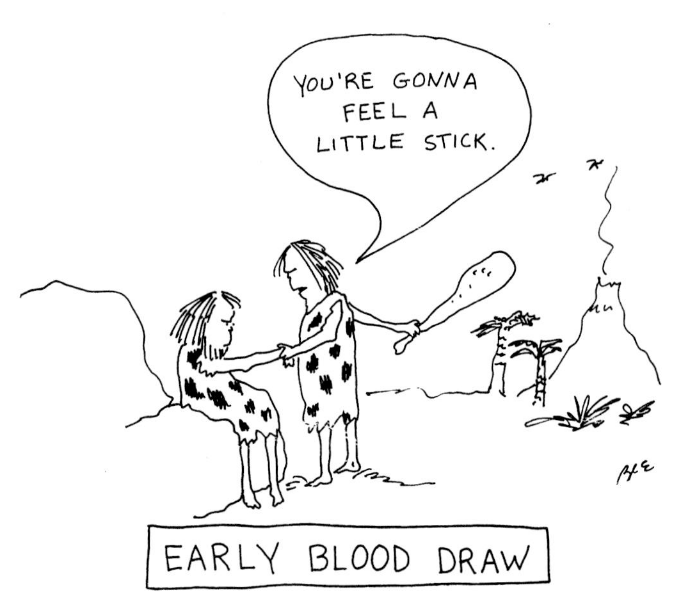

2.

Between a Doc and a Scarred Place

You've got me in stitches

Ticklish operations

Oops!

Surgery on the fly

Surgery for the faint-hearted

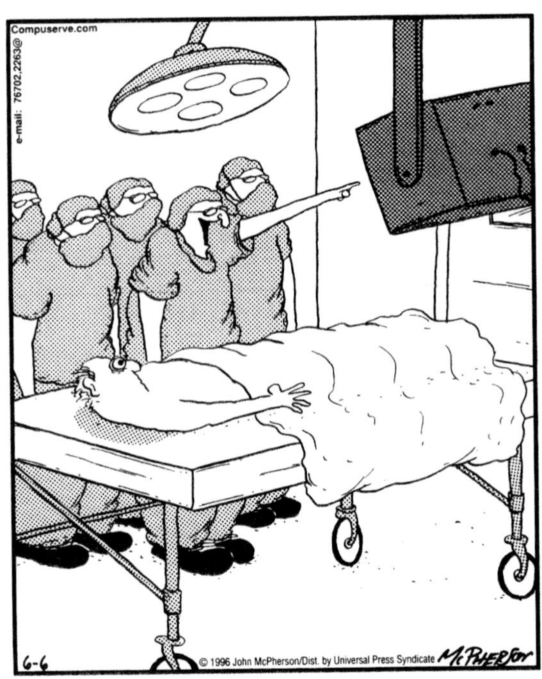

"Stop the tape! See what George Clooney is doing with that catheter? That's the procedure I think we should try with Mr. Simkins."

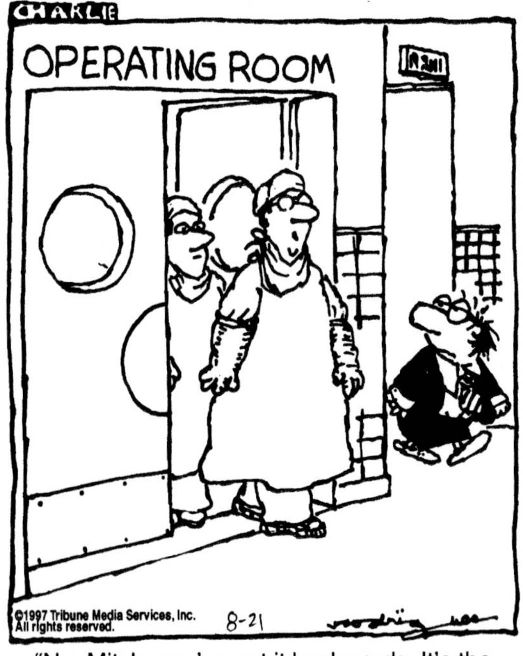

"No, Mitch, you've got it backwards. It's the Lexus LS400 that's three double-bypasses, not the Mercedes-Benz S600.

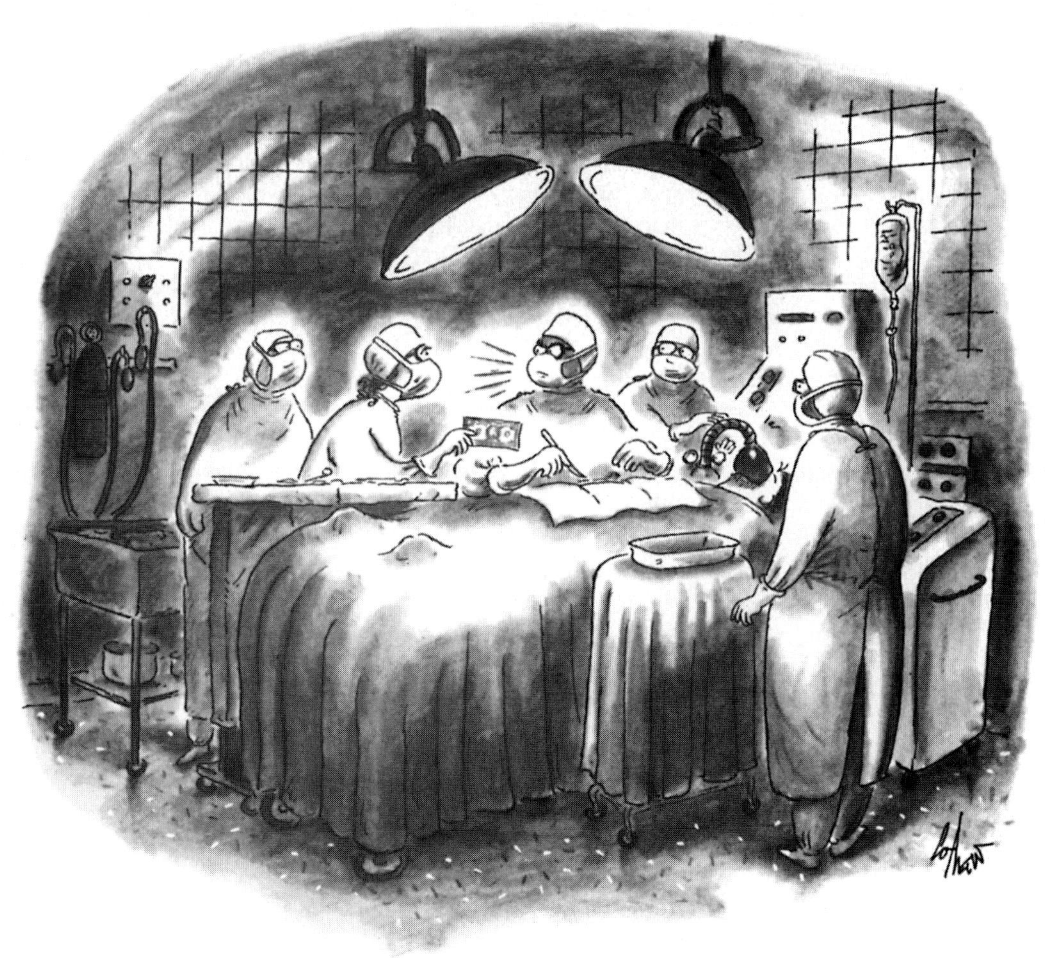

"Damn it, nurse! I didn't ask for a twenty. I asked for a ten and two fives."

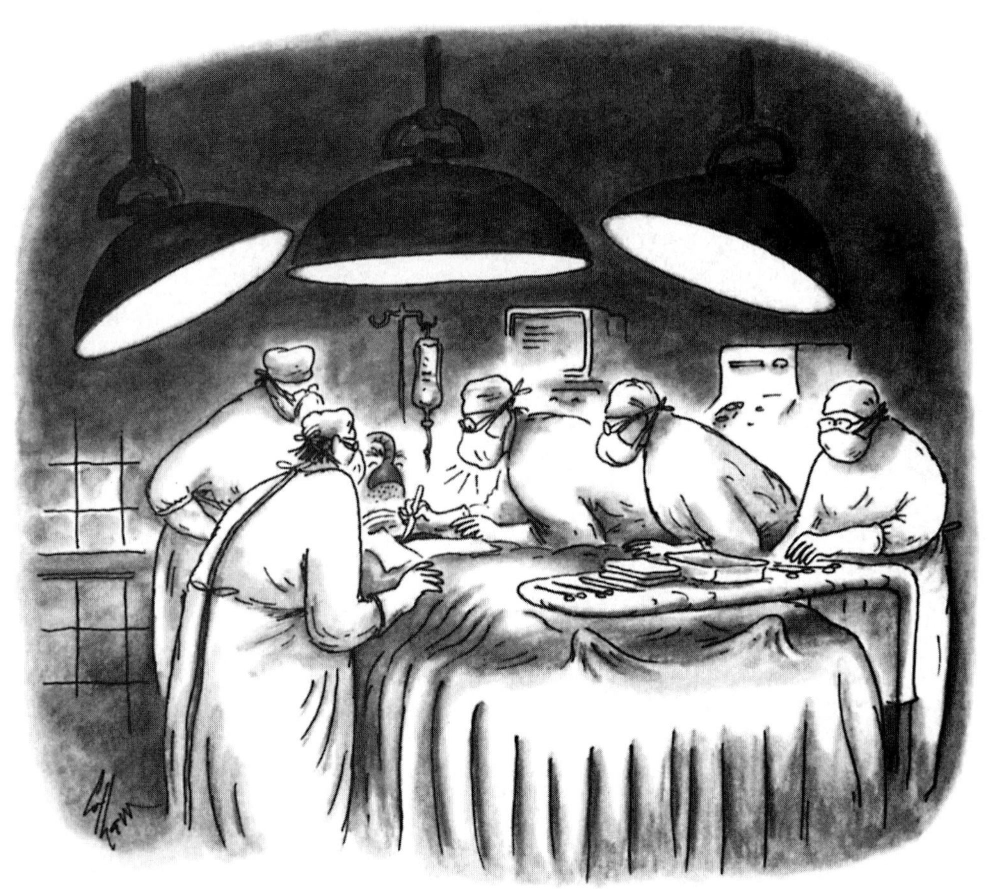

"Hey, I've operated on this guy before—there are my initials."

Nick Downes

MOORE
YO, HIGGINS! YOU'D BETTER START WARMING UP...
12-24

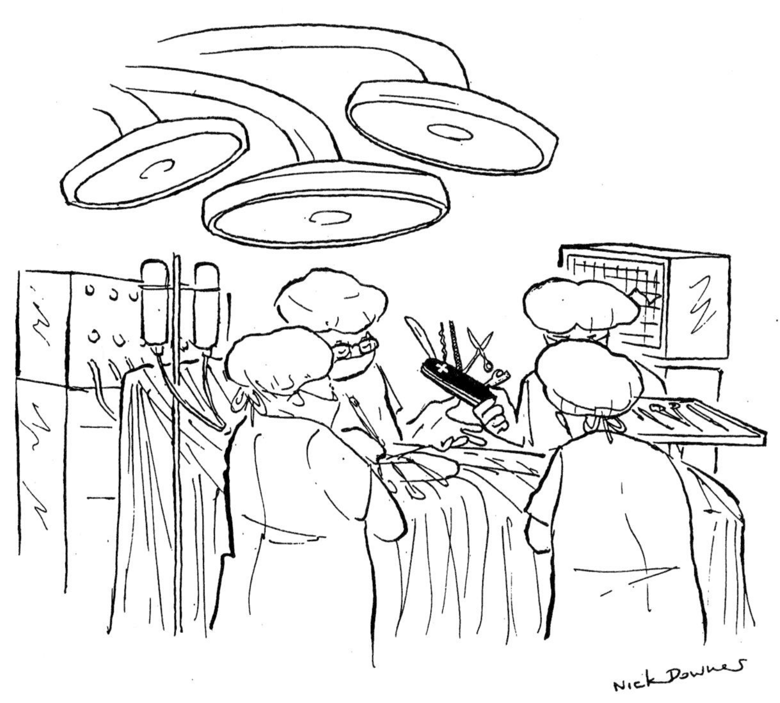

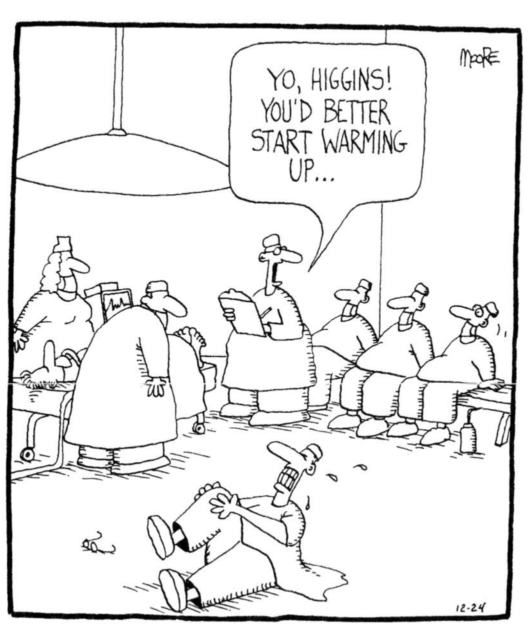

Halfway though gall bladder surgery, Dr. Wilson fakes left, cuts right and goes down with a knee injury.

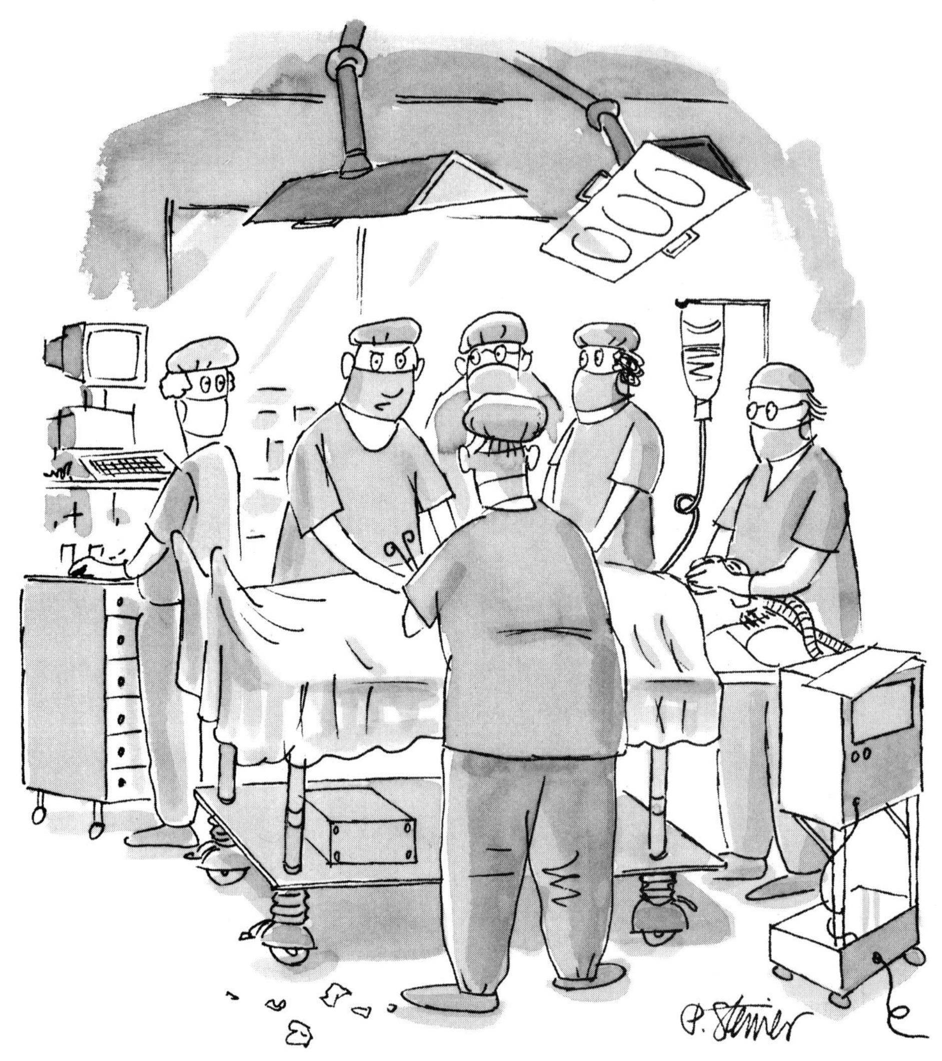

"Hey, c'mon. This isn't brain surgery."

CHARLIE
X-RAY 1
MEN
HEART SURGEONS MUST WASH HANDS!
10-18
©1997 Tribune Media Services, Inc.
All rights reserved.

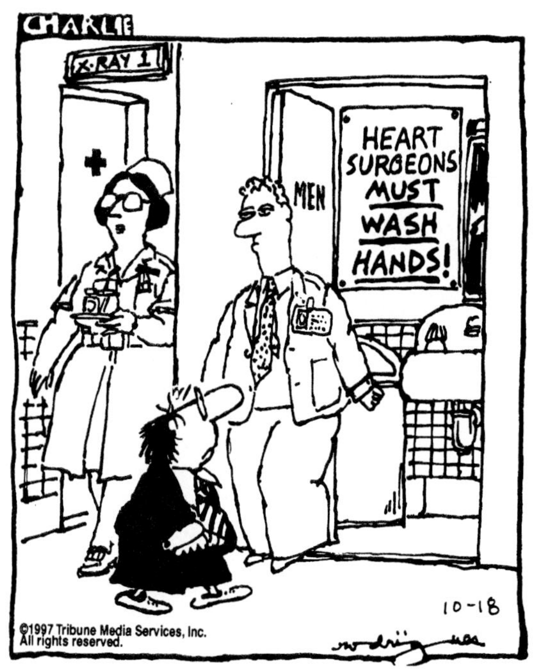

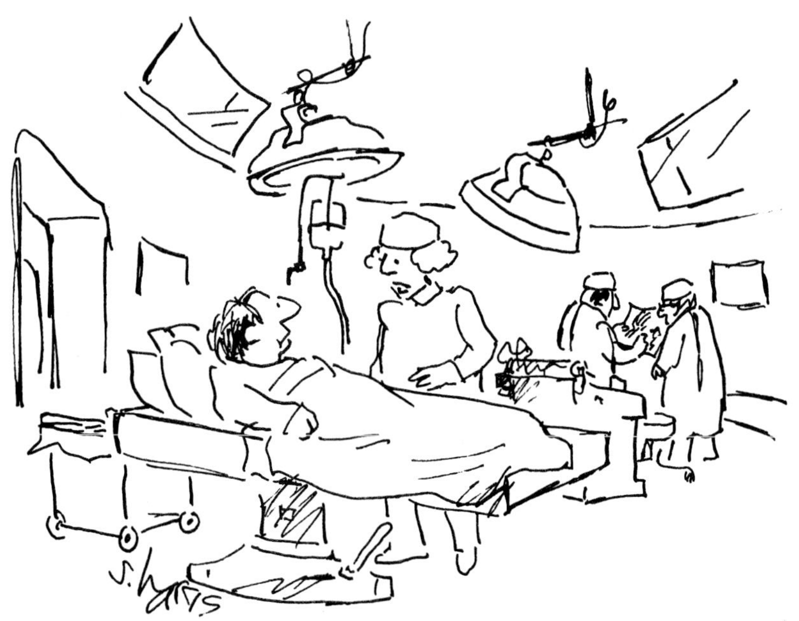

"You'll find that what the Doctor lacks in technique, he makes up in warmth and sincerity."

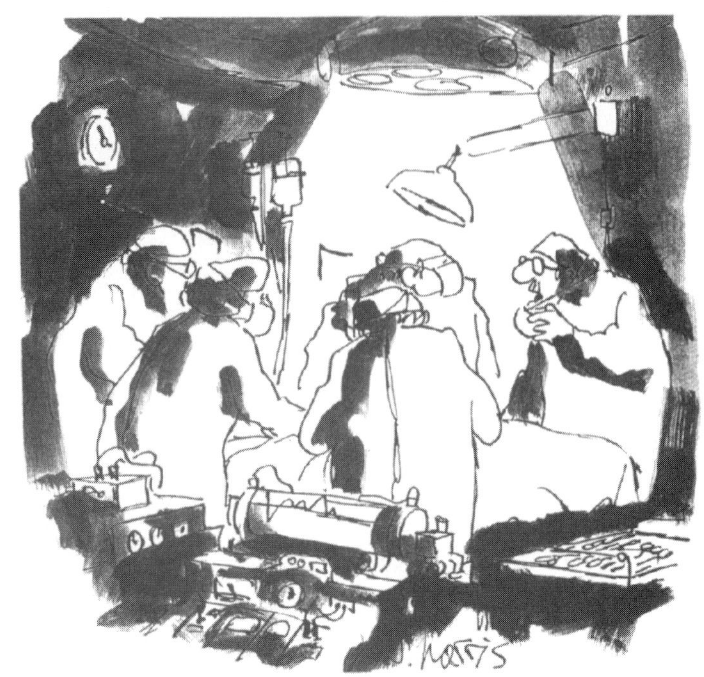

"Anyone here who didn't take the hippocratic Oath?"

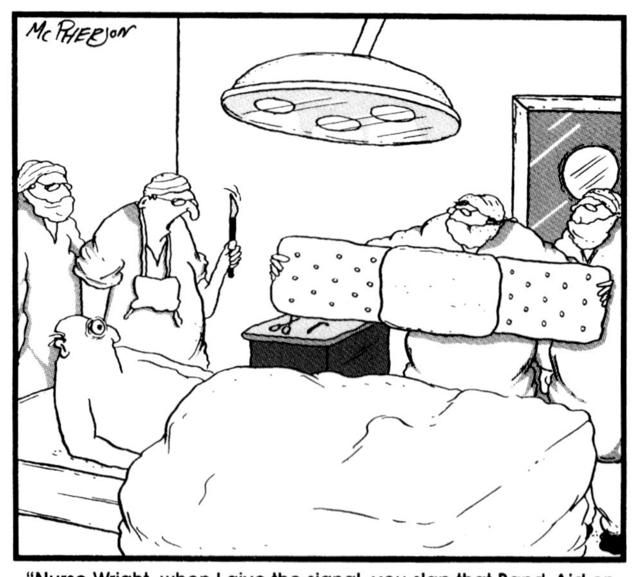

"Nurse Wright, when I give the signal, you slap that Band-Aid on him as fast as possible."

IN THE BLEACHERS By Steve Moore

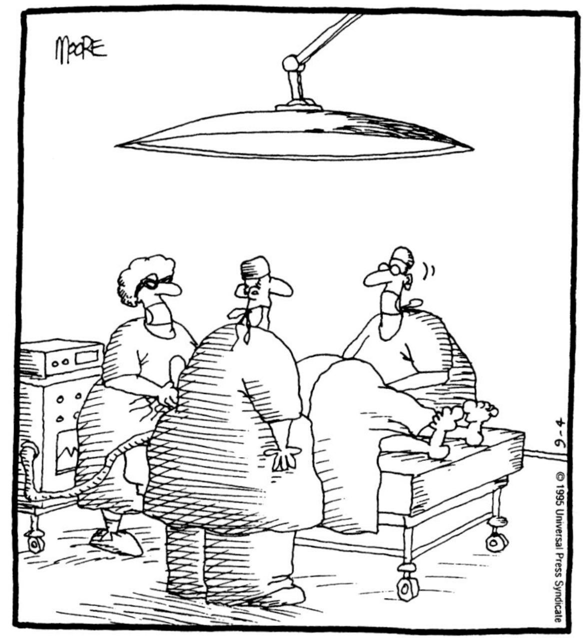

"Well, we can't just say that we removed 'a big growth.' It's gotta be dramatic ... Is it the size of a volleyball, soccer ball or basketball?"

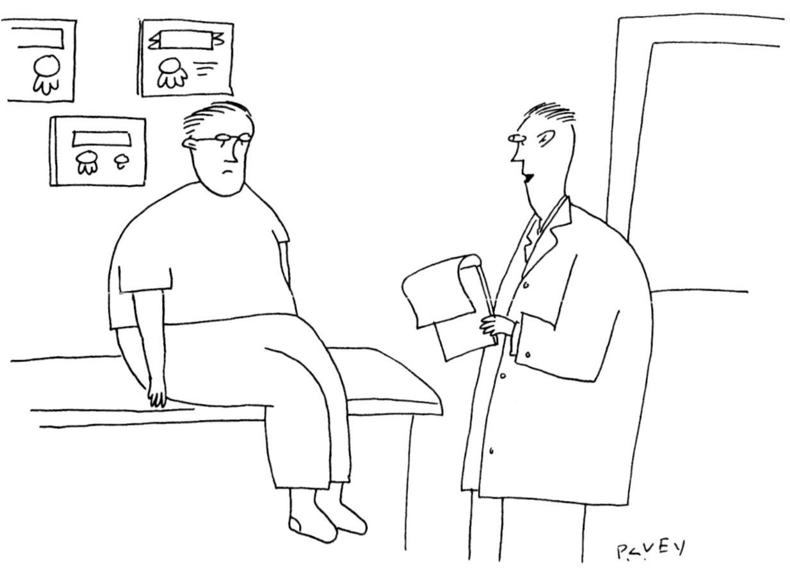

"Three words, Mr. Fitzpatrick, unnecessary brain surgery."

YOURS IS A VERY SIMPLE OPERATION MR. YATES. WE JUST OPEN THE SKULL RIGHT HERE AND... IM SORRY. WHAT WAS I SAYING?
McLAREN

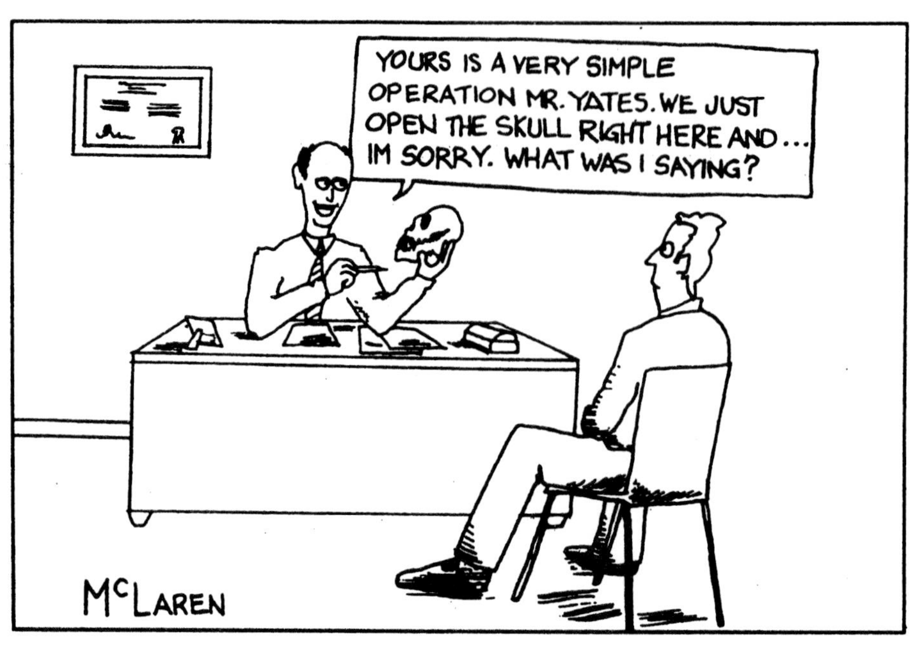

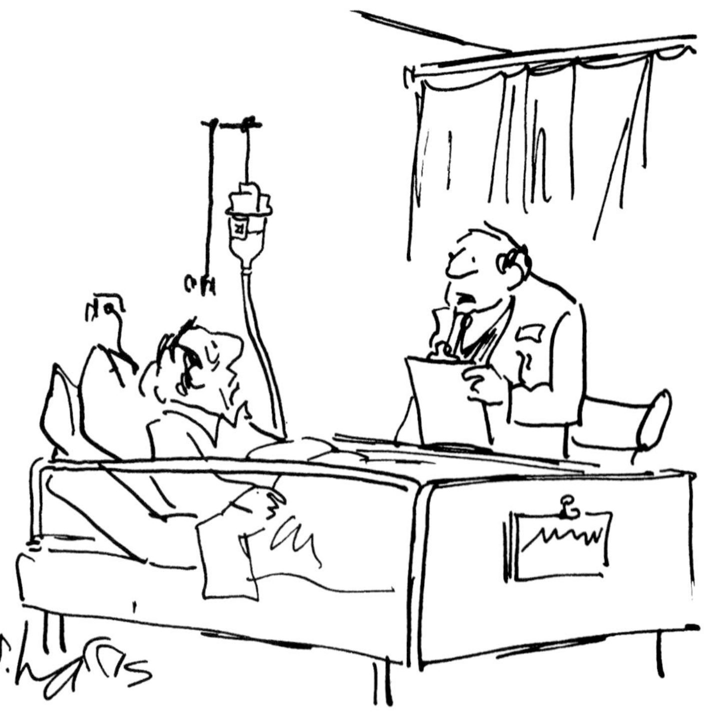

"We sincerely regret the unnecessary surgery, and we're going to put back as much as we possibly can."

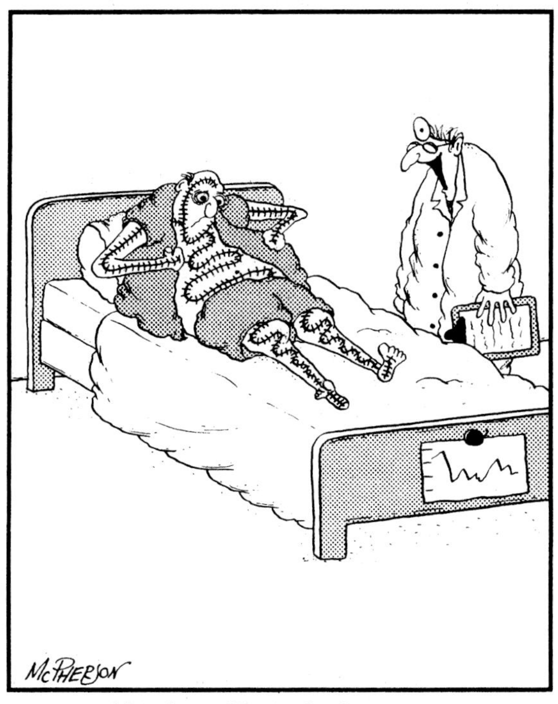

"Good news! The exploratory surgery turned up negative!"

IN THE BLEACHERS By Steve Moore

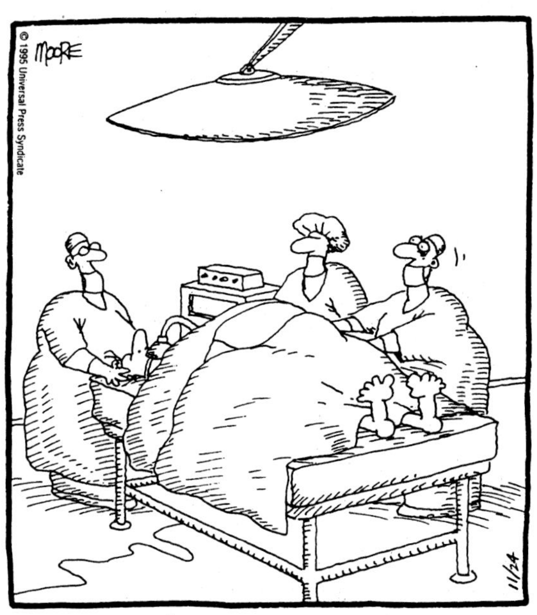

"I KNOW the procedure is running long, Dr. Markovich. But quit referring to it as 'sudden-death overtime.'"

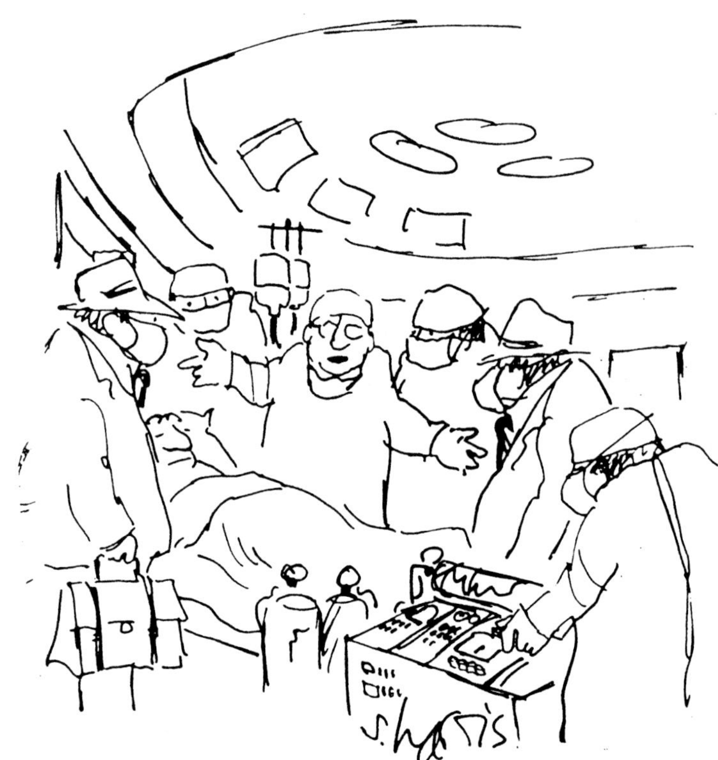

"All right, now — the patient's lawyer will stand on the right side, and our lawyer will stand on the left side."

HERMAN®

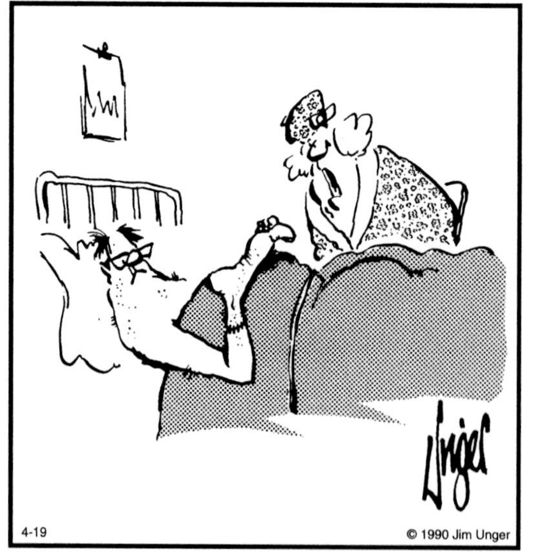

"My cousin, Irene, knows a good lawyer."

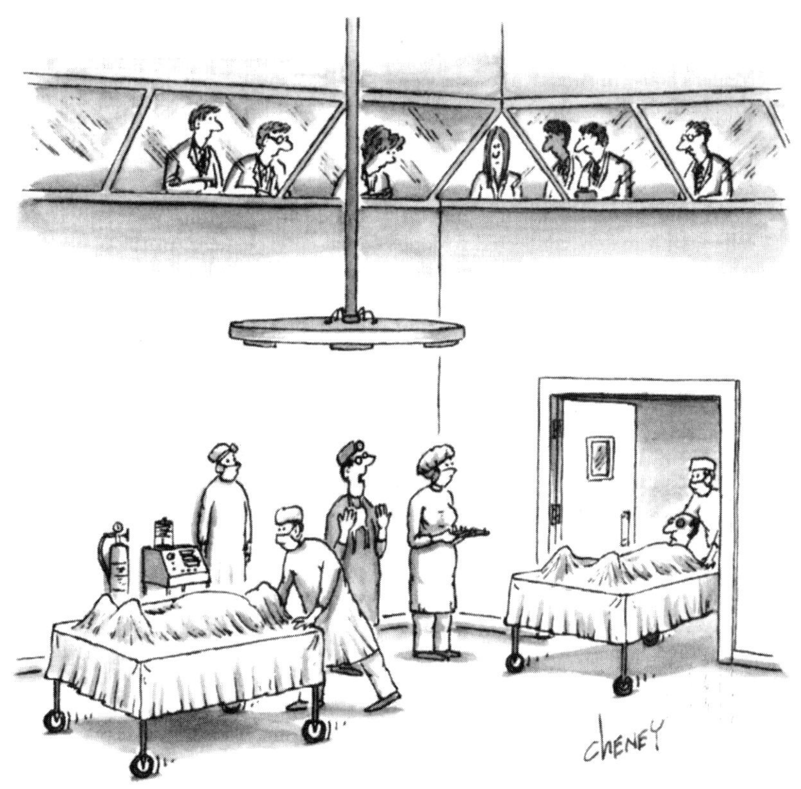

"Next, an example of the very same procedure when done correctly."

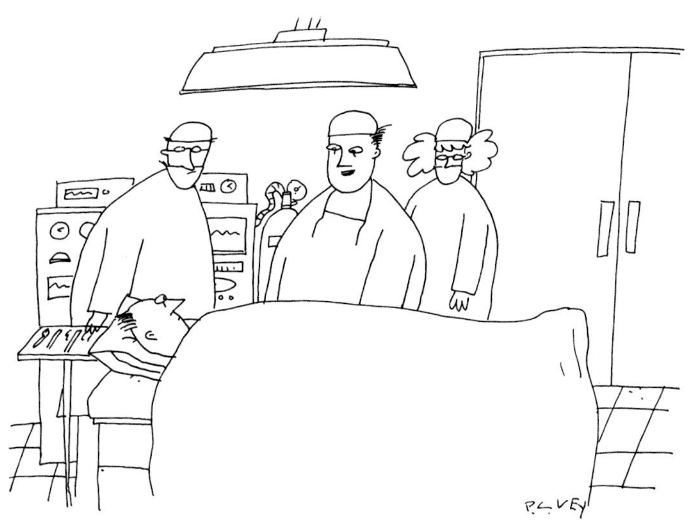

"I've decided to play God today, I hope you don't mind."

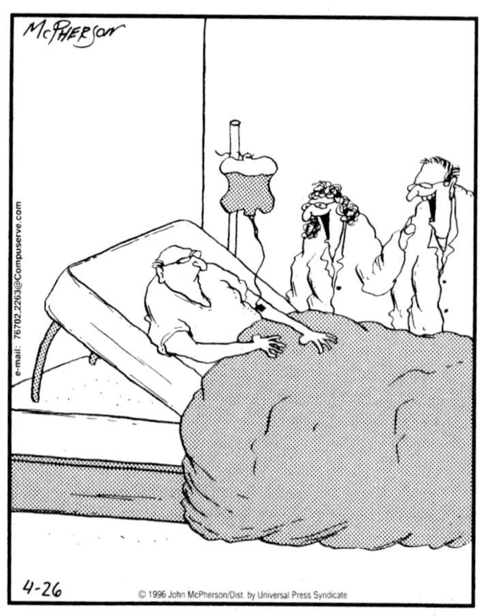

"Good news, Mr. Duffman! You're not crazy after all. You *have* been hearing voices coming from your abdomen. We discovered that Dr. Gremley's pager accidentally got sutured inside you during surgery!"

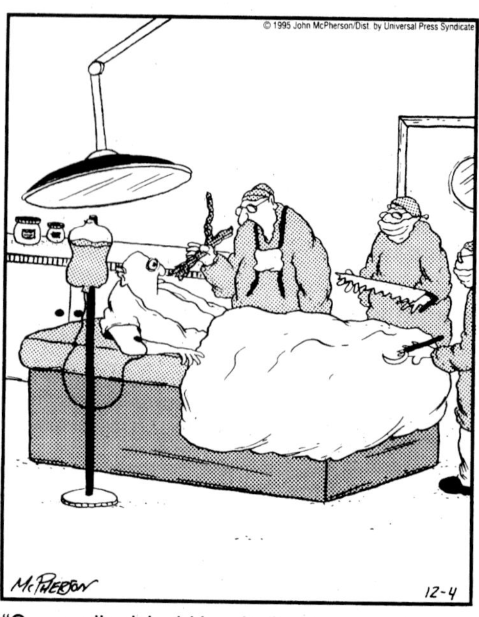

"Our anesthesiologist is out with a head cold. When I say 'now,' bite on this stick as hard as you can."

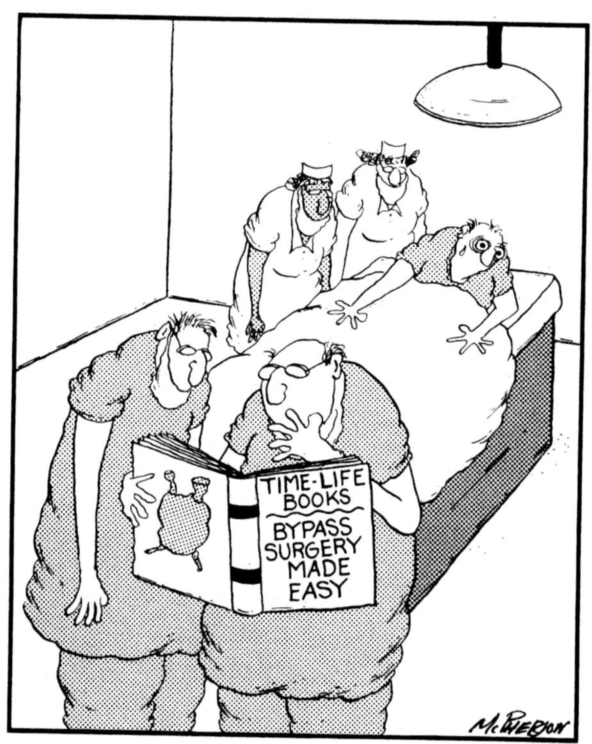

3.

On the Couch

Mind over matter

I'm not paranoid am I?

Strange sagas from the psychiatrist's office

Let's analyze this

THE FAR SIDE By GARY LARSON

© 1990 FarWorks, Inc./Dist. by Universal Press Syndi
Just plain nuts!
3-13

HOW TO FEEL GOOD
HOW TO FEEL GREAT

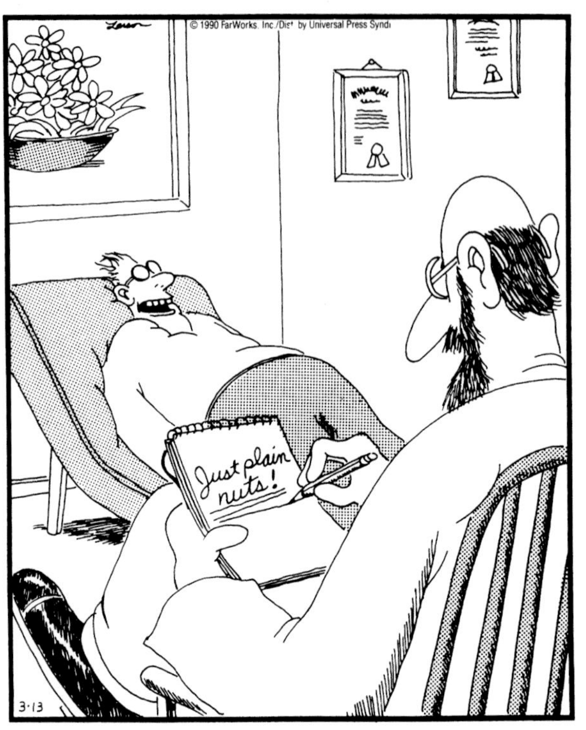

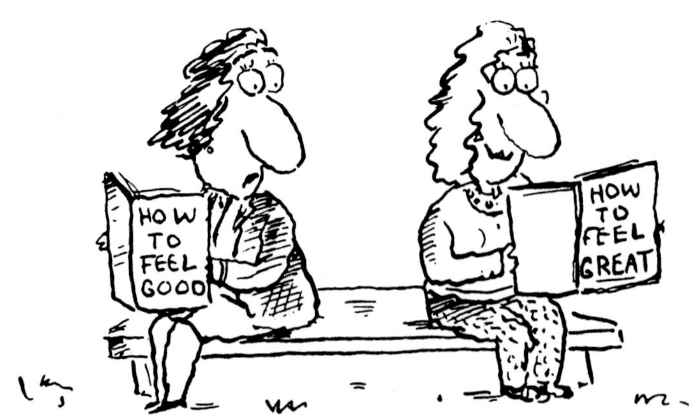

SIPRESS

...so I said, "Hold on Doc, later for the family therapy. Let's just put the whole kit n'kaboodle on anti-depressants!"
SIPRESS

Farcus
by David Waisglass
Gordon Coulthart
© 1992 Farcus Cartoons
WAISGLASS/COULTHART

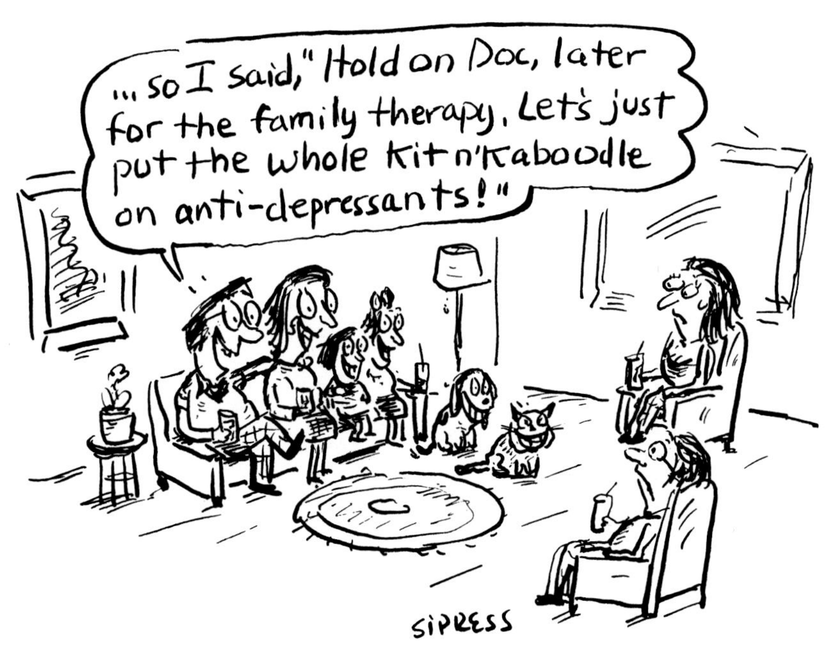

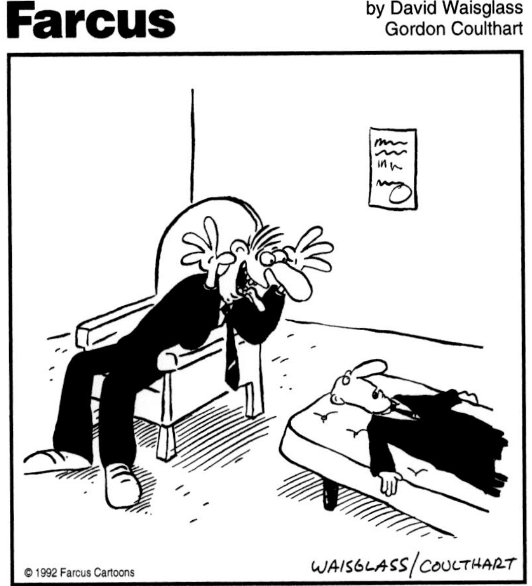

"Call me paranoid, but I think people at work are making fun of me."

MANKOFF

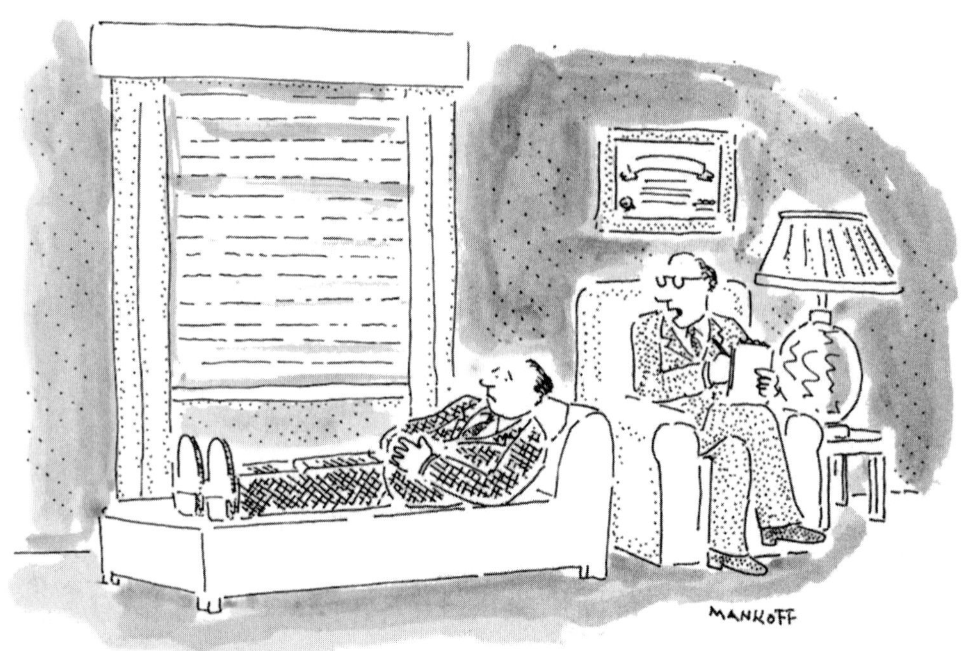

"Why don't you just go and see this summer's feel-good movie?"

YOU'RE A FAILURE
YOU'RE A LOSER
YOU'LL NEVER AMOUNT TO ANYTHING
It's a motivational technique I learned from my father.
SIPRESS

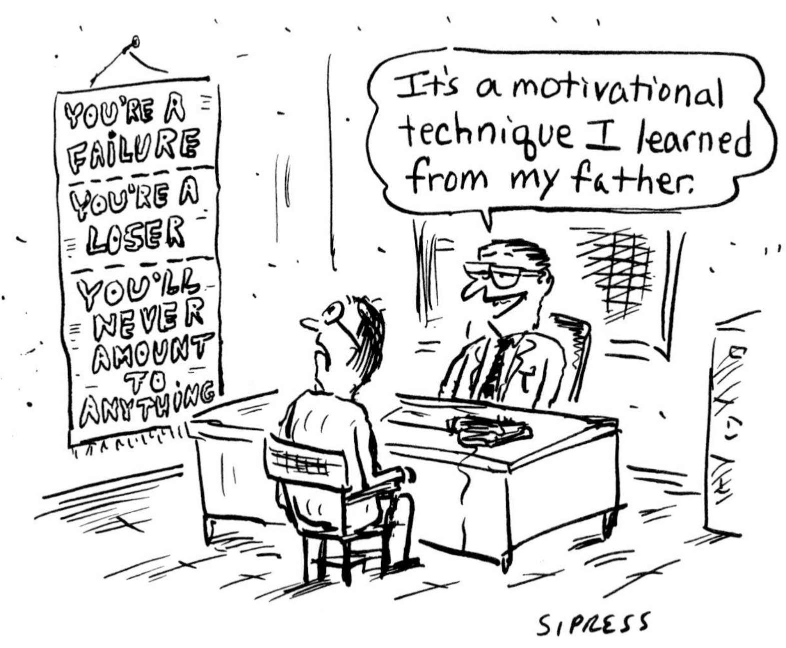

IN THE BLEACHERS

By Steve Moore

JdsmooRe@AoL.com
© 1996 Universal Press Syndicate
...AND CARL MAKES A GRUNTING NOISE WHEN HE SWINGS.
OH, OK. LET'S TALK ABOUT ANNOYING SOUNDS, MR. CHRONIC STOMACH GAS!
THEY NEVER LET ME DRIVE THE CART.
PLEASE STOP YELLING!!
KLEENEX
9-16 MOORE

Golf foursome in counseling.

I'M SORRY, I CANNOT CONTINUE THIS SESSION! YOU'RE JUST LIKE MY FATHER WHO USED TO LIE AROUND ON THE COUCH ALL DAY COMPLAINING! GET A JOB, YOU WORM!
5·18
PIRARO ©DAN PIRARO 1995· DIST. BY UNIVERSAL PRESS SYND. E·MAIL: BIZARRO95@AOL.COM

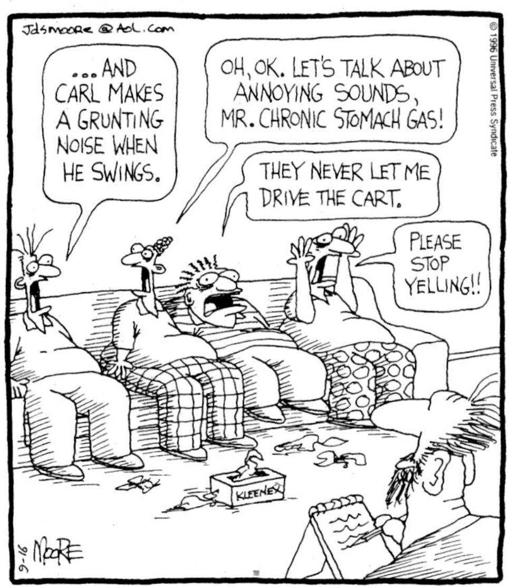

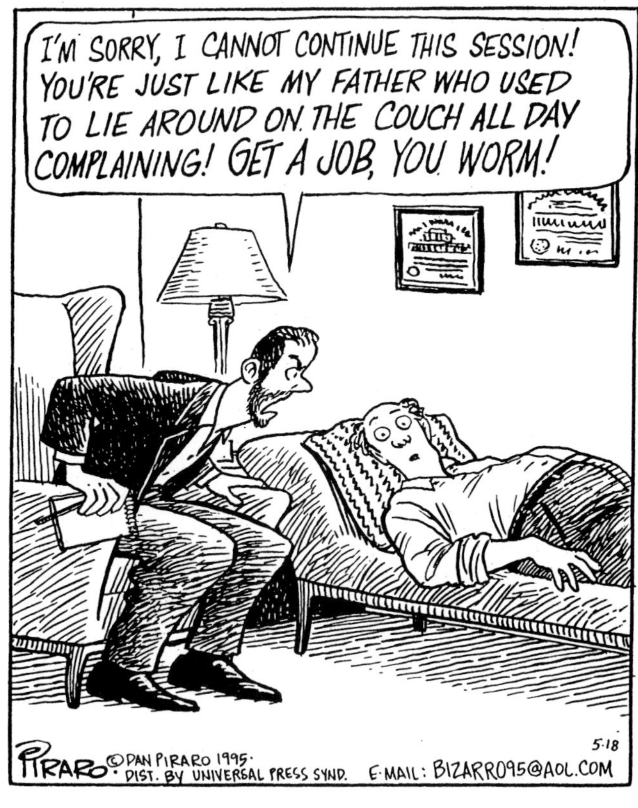

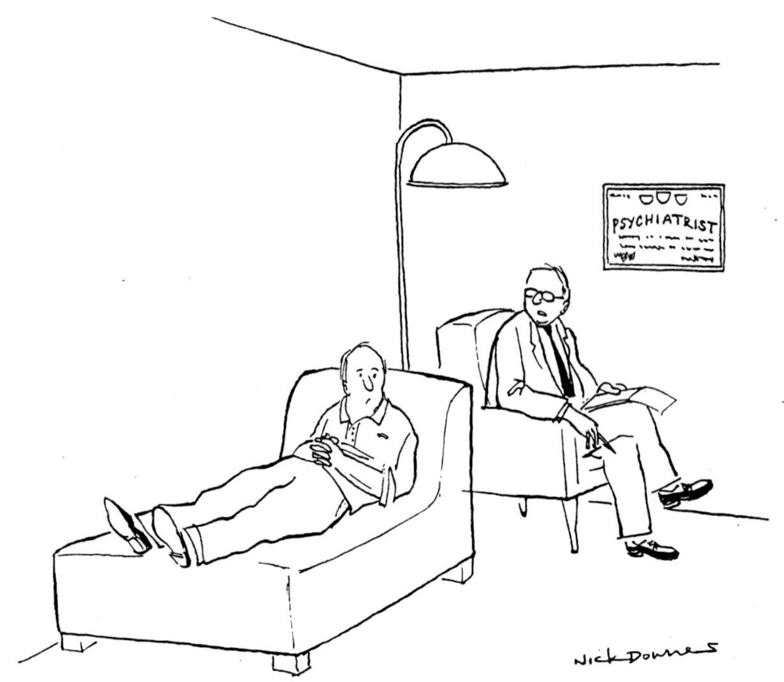

"It's wrong to consider yourself a loser, Mr. Conley. Rather, think of yourself as an enabler of others to win."

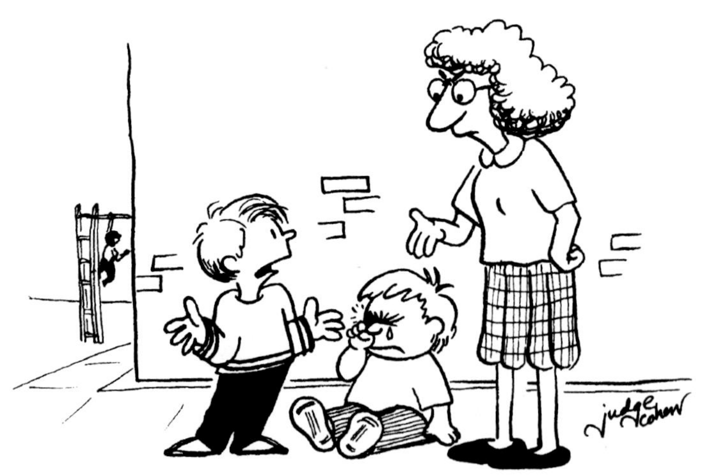

"I couldn't help myself. My lack of serotonin made me do it."

RIVERDALE MENTAL HEALTH CLINIC
I'D RATHER BE DEAD
I BRAKE FOR HALLUCINATIONS
MY OTHER CAR HAS A HOSE HOOKED UP TO THE EXHAUST
NICK DOWNES

S. Harris

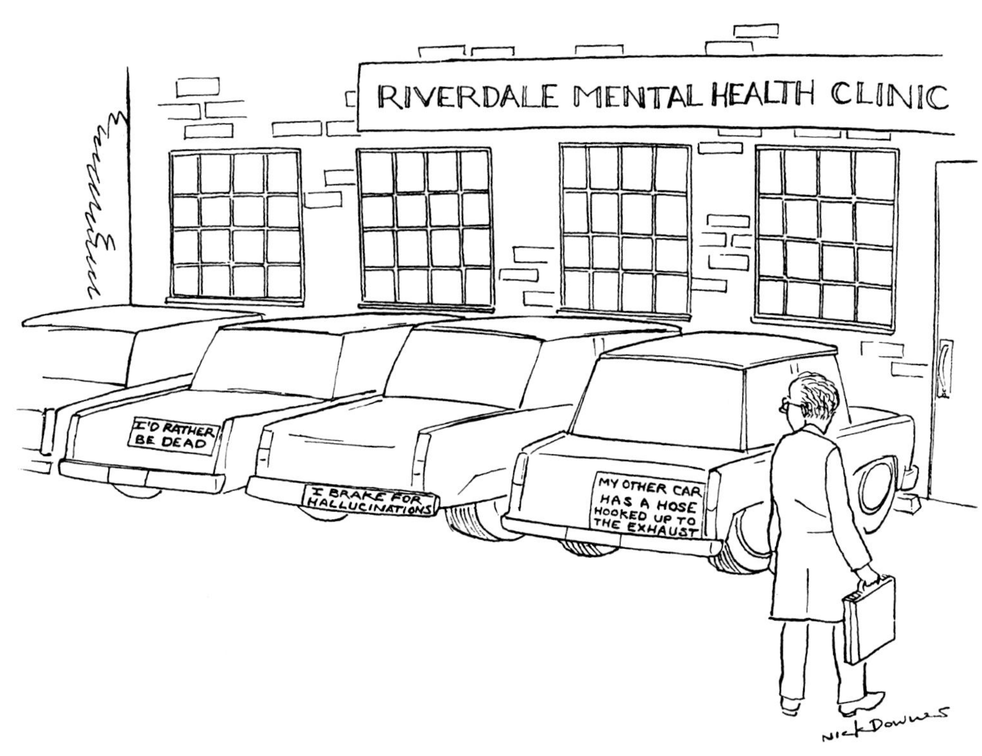

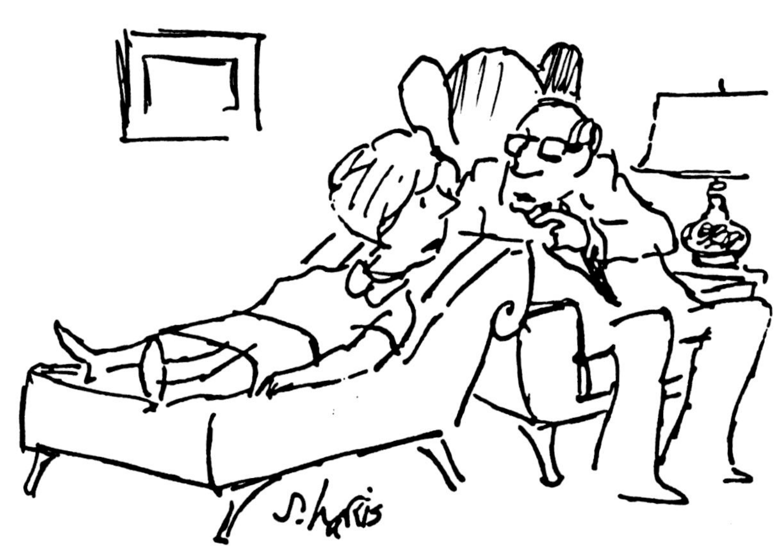

"Stick to your obsessions. Your compulsions aren't covered by your insurance plan."

ADVANCED 12-STEP:

I am currently able to take it one milli-second at a time...
SIPRESS © 97

PSYCHIATRIST
BILL HARRISON

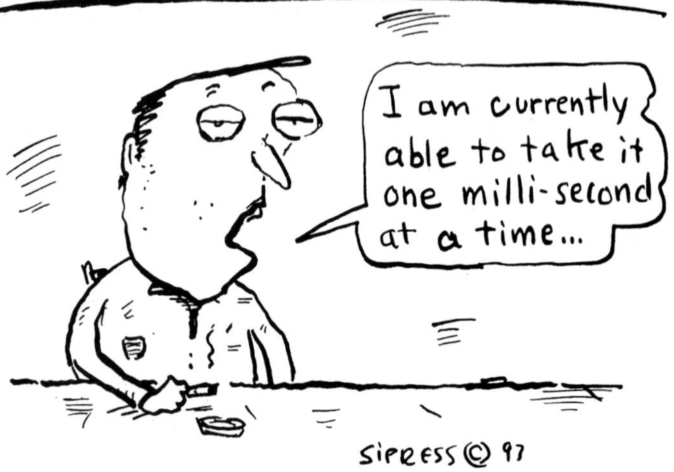

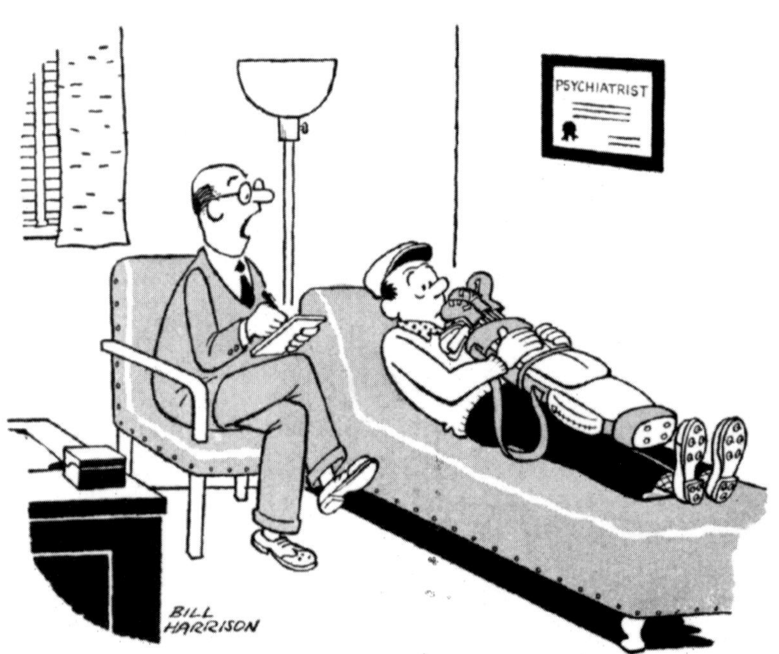

"You need something to take your mind off your hobby."

CBarsotti

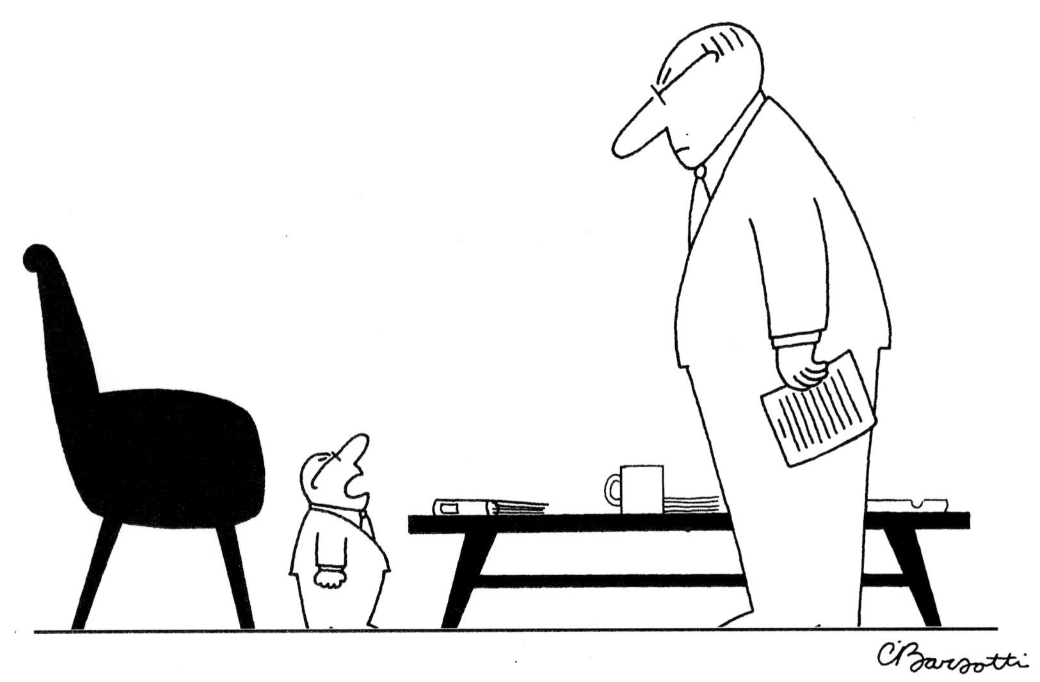

"Yeah? Well, I've heard this Napoleonic complex stuff all my life, pal, and I'm sick of it."

...and now, on top of everything else, I've got the guilt about making people sick...
SIPRESS© 86

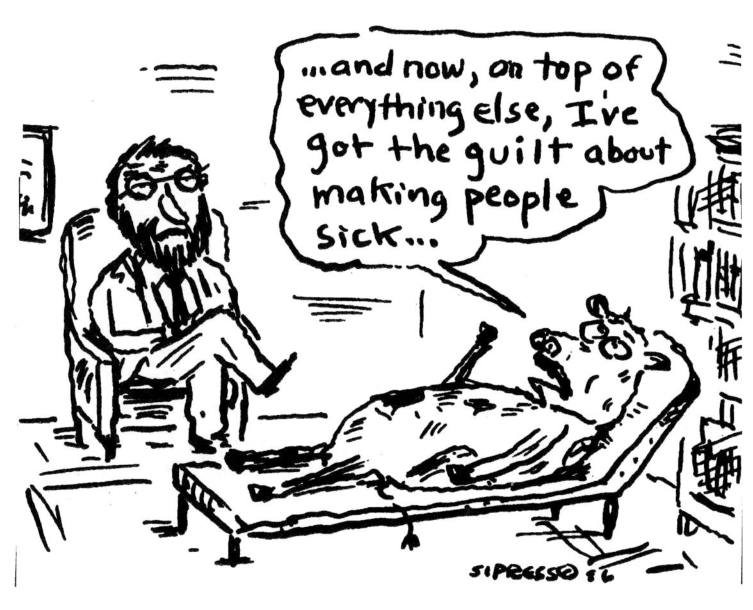

BOY, I FEEL
HORRIBLE
MCLAREN

Post Possum Depression

I've called this meeting to discuss the problem of stress in the workplace!
SIPRESS

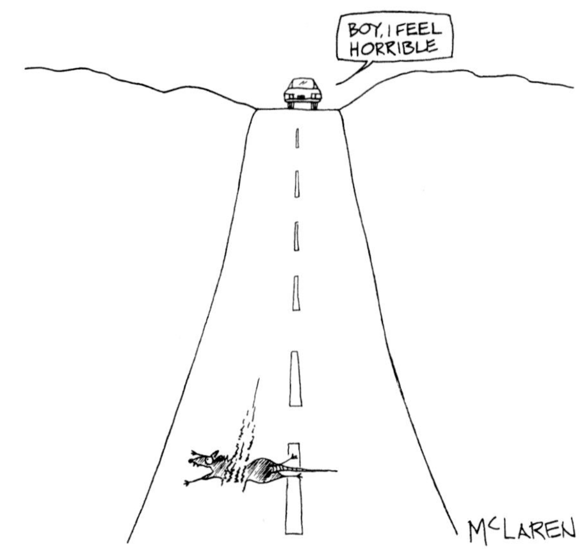

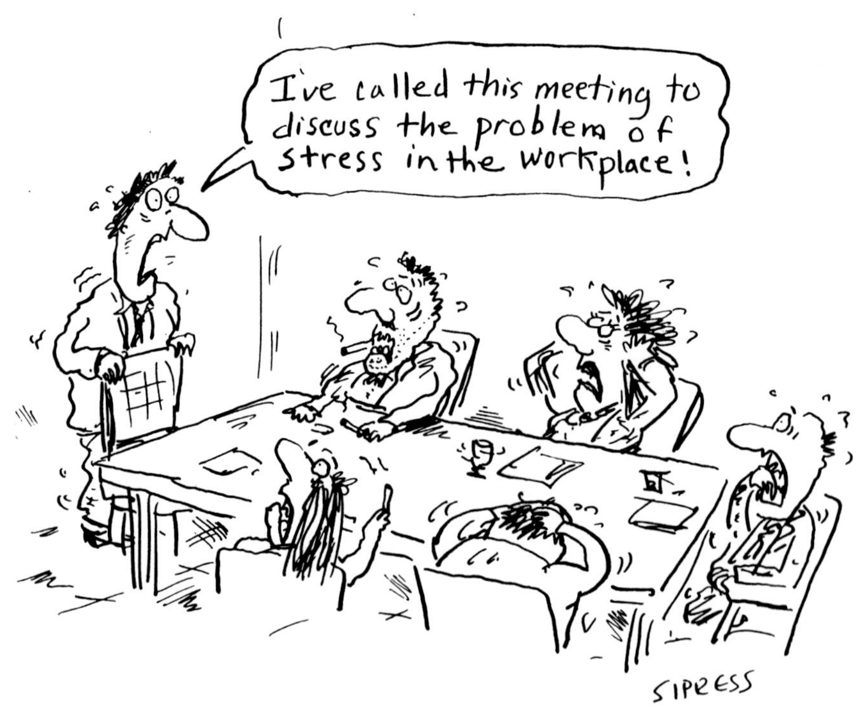

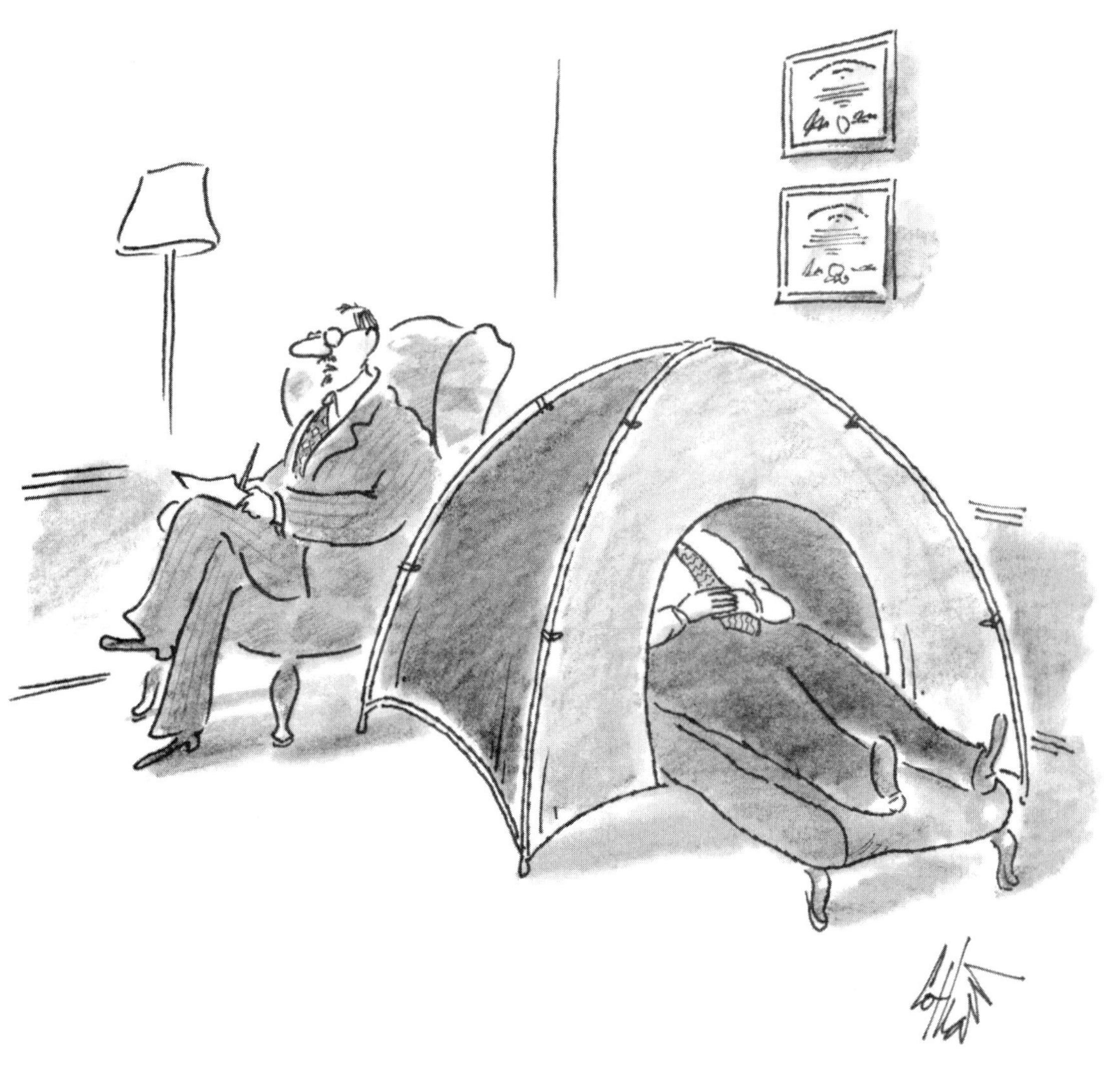

"I understand that you are not a happy camper."

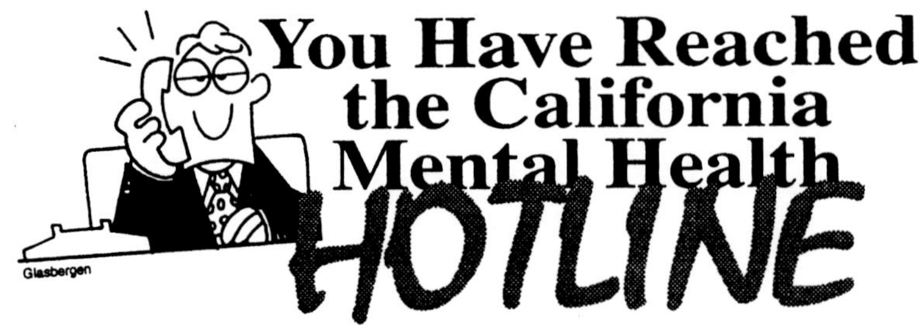

• If you are obsessive-compulsive, press 1 over and over and over again;

• If you are multiple personality, touch 3, 4, 5, 6, 7, and 8;

• If you are hysterical, don't touch any buttons whatsoever, something terrible might happen;

• If you are bipolar, touch 1, then 9;

• If you are schizophrenic, don't touch any buttons, a little voice will tell you what to do;

• If you are a paranoid, there is no need to touch any buttons, we know who you are, we know where you live, and we will be coming to get you very soon;

• If you are a psychopath, rip the cord out of the wall, and run away with the phone;

• If you are an anal-retentive psychopath, take the phone apart. Place each piece in a plastic bag. Tape each plastic bag tightly shut. Place all the plastic bags into a large, brown paper bag, which you then place in the southeast corner of your freezer.

• If you are depressed, do not touch any buttons, it wouldn't do any good anyway;

• If you are manic, touch as many buttons as you can as fast as possible;

• If you are a narcissist, touch yourself.

Contributed by Don Schwartz

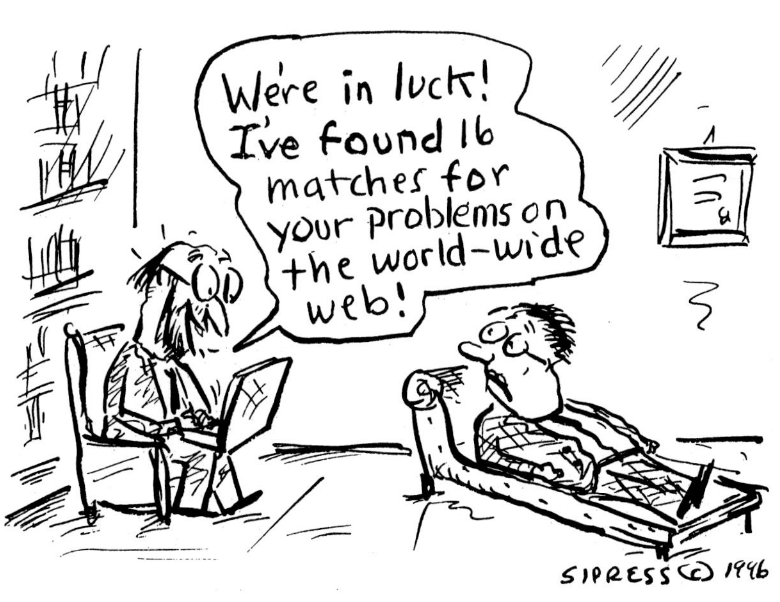
We're in luck! I've found 16 matches for your problems on the world-wide web!
SIPRESS © 1996

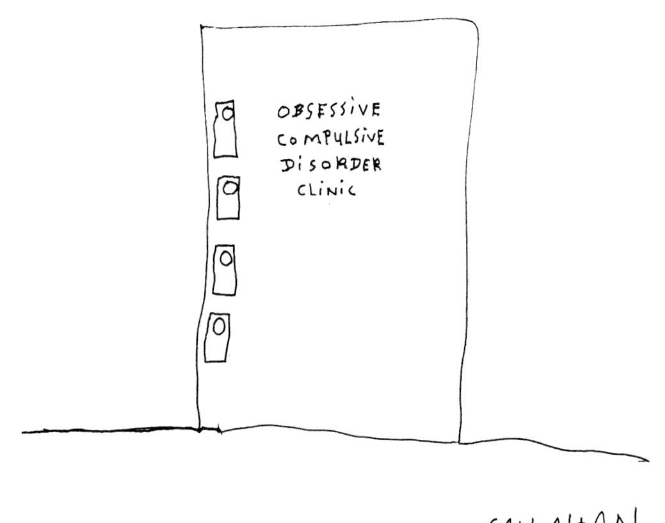
OBSESSIVE
COMPULSIVE
DISORDER
CLINIC
CALLAHAN

"Lite" Psychiatry
SIPRESS © 1990
Why don't we talk about what you're going to wear Saturday night?

S. Harris

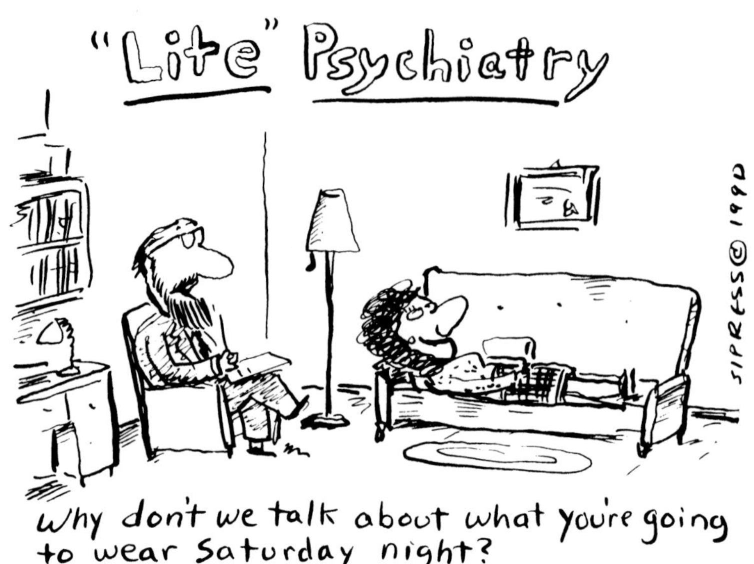

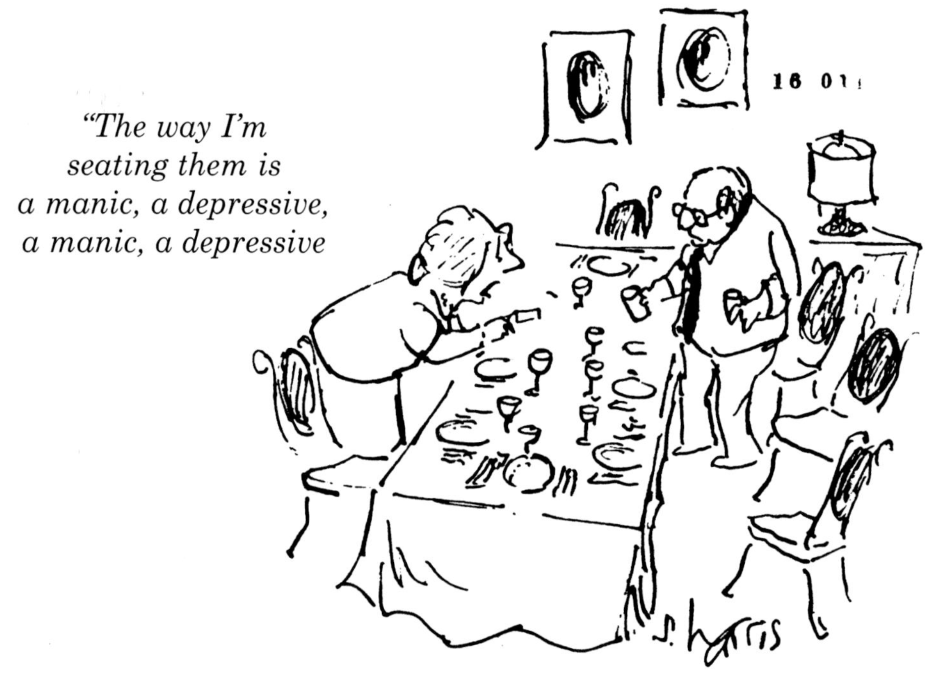

"The way I'm seating them is a manic, a depressive, a manic, a depressive

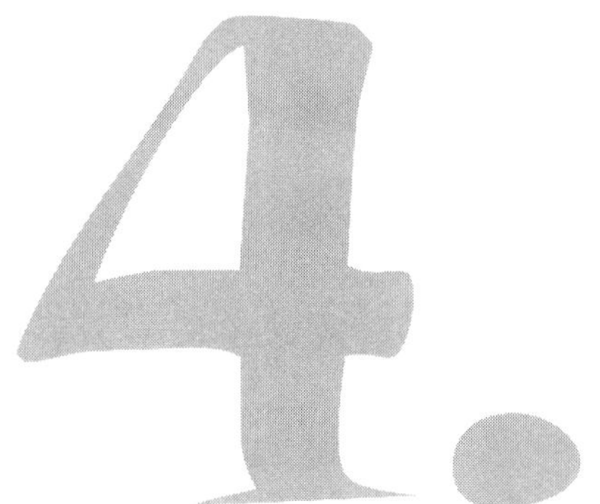

Within Humorous Limits

Laughter is the best medicine

Diseases that defy definition

Medical predicaments

Bizarre hospital encounters

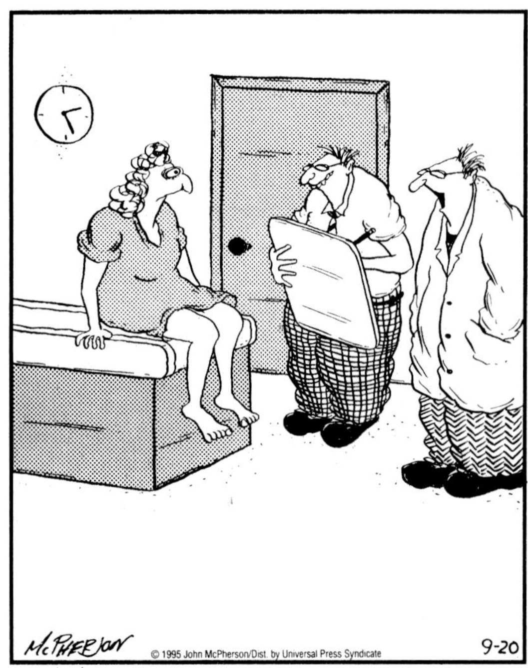

"Unfortunately, Mrs. Dortford, our entire X-ray department is on strike. But if you'll just describe your pain in as much detail as possible, our staff sketch artist should be able to give us a fairly accurate drawing of the problem."

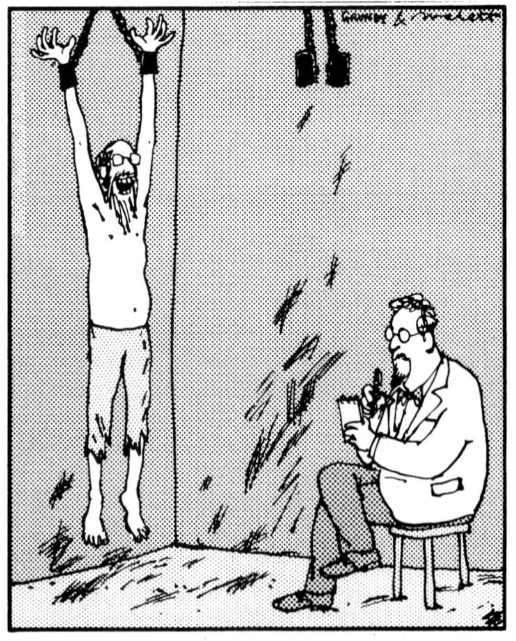

"Call me weird, but I feel good!"

Adam® by Brian Basset

NOW THEN, LET'S CHECK YOUR REFLEXES.
"GRAPE POPSICLE"
CLAYTON! KATY! NOT IN THE LIVING ROOM AND ESPECIALLY NOT ON THE GOOD COUCH!
EXCELLENT!
© 1993 Universal Press Syndicate
BRIAN BASSET
1-7

HERMAN®

5-26
© 1988 Jim Unger
Unger

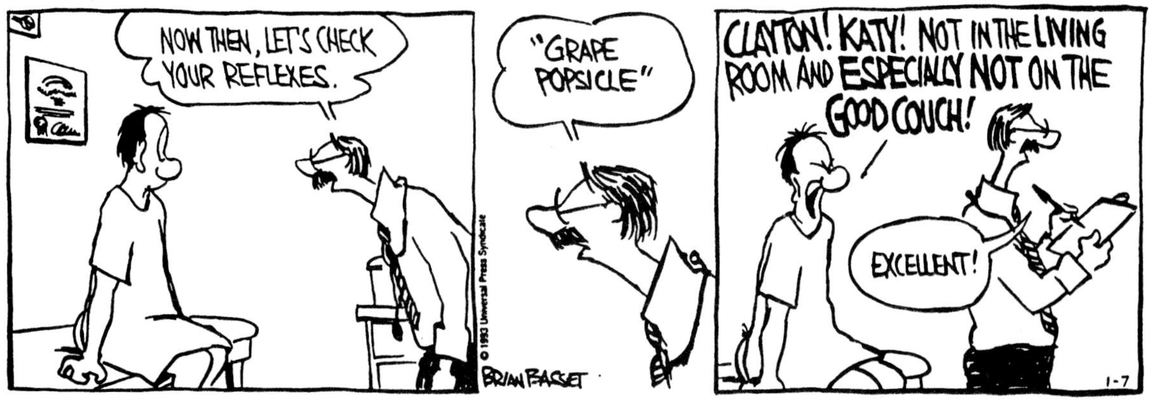

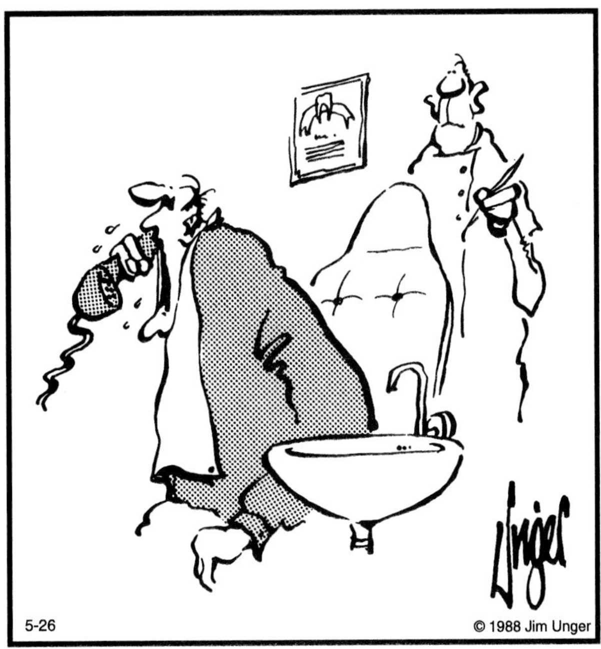

"I'b spled, I'b spill ab de benpisp."

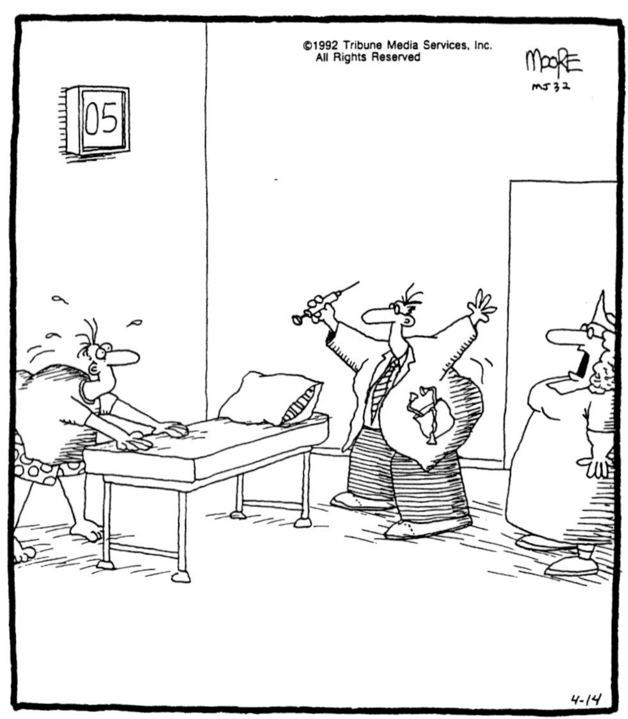

"Hurry, doctor! Only five seconds left on the shot clock!!"

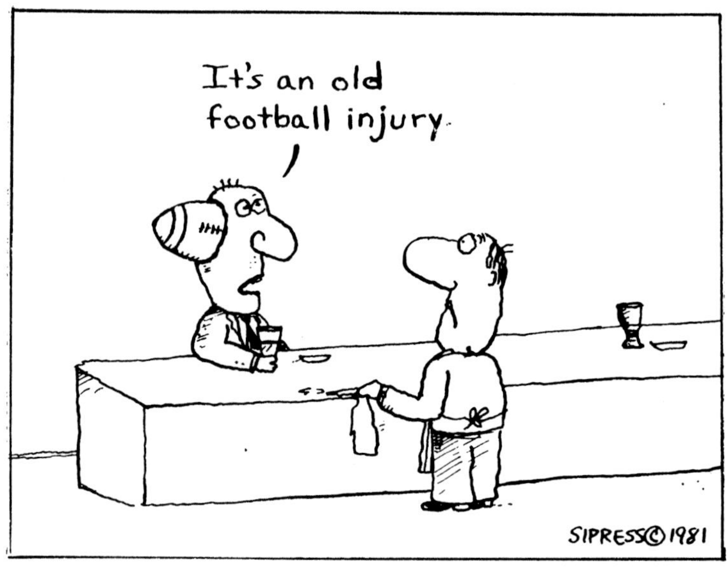

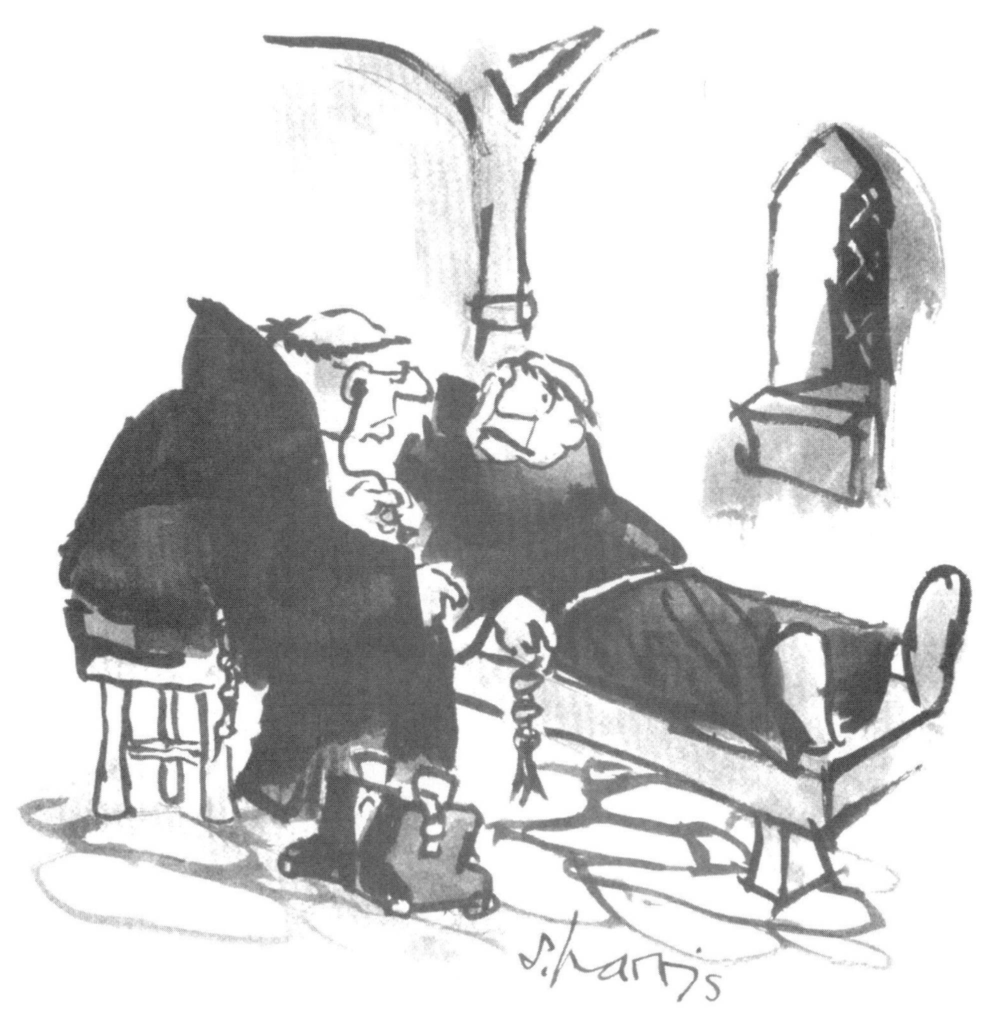

"What do you mean 'Don't expect miracles'?
why shouldn't I expect miracles?"

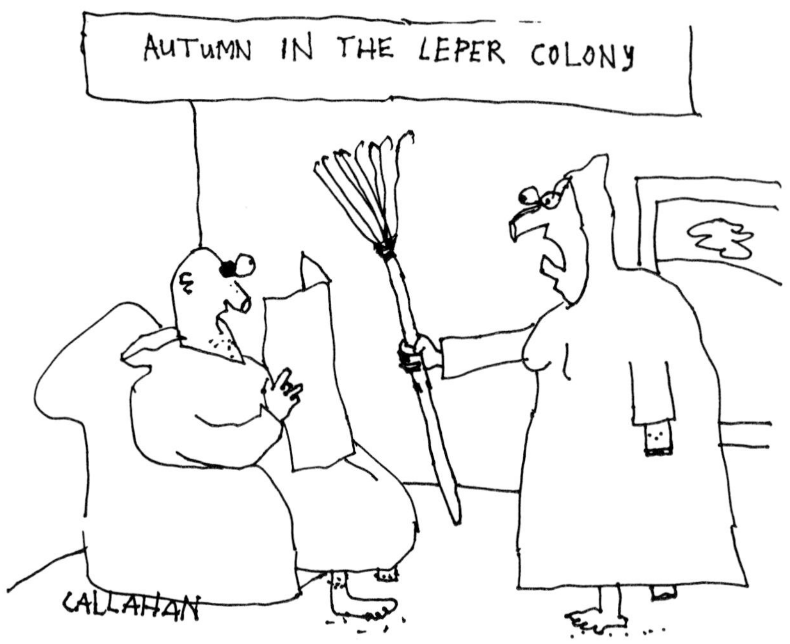

"Now get out there and rake up those fallen limbs!"

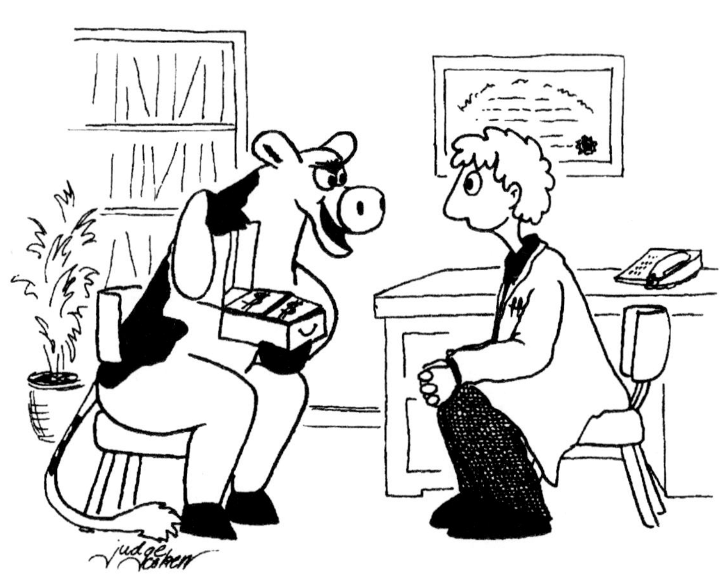

"...and if your research just happens to prove beef is carcinogenic, there'll be plenty more where *this* came from."

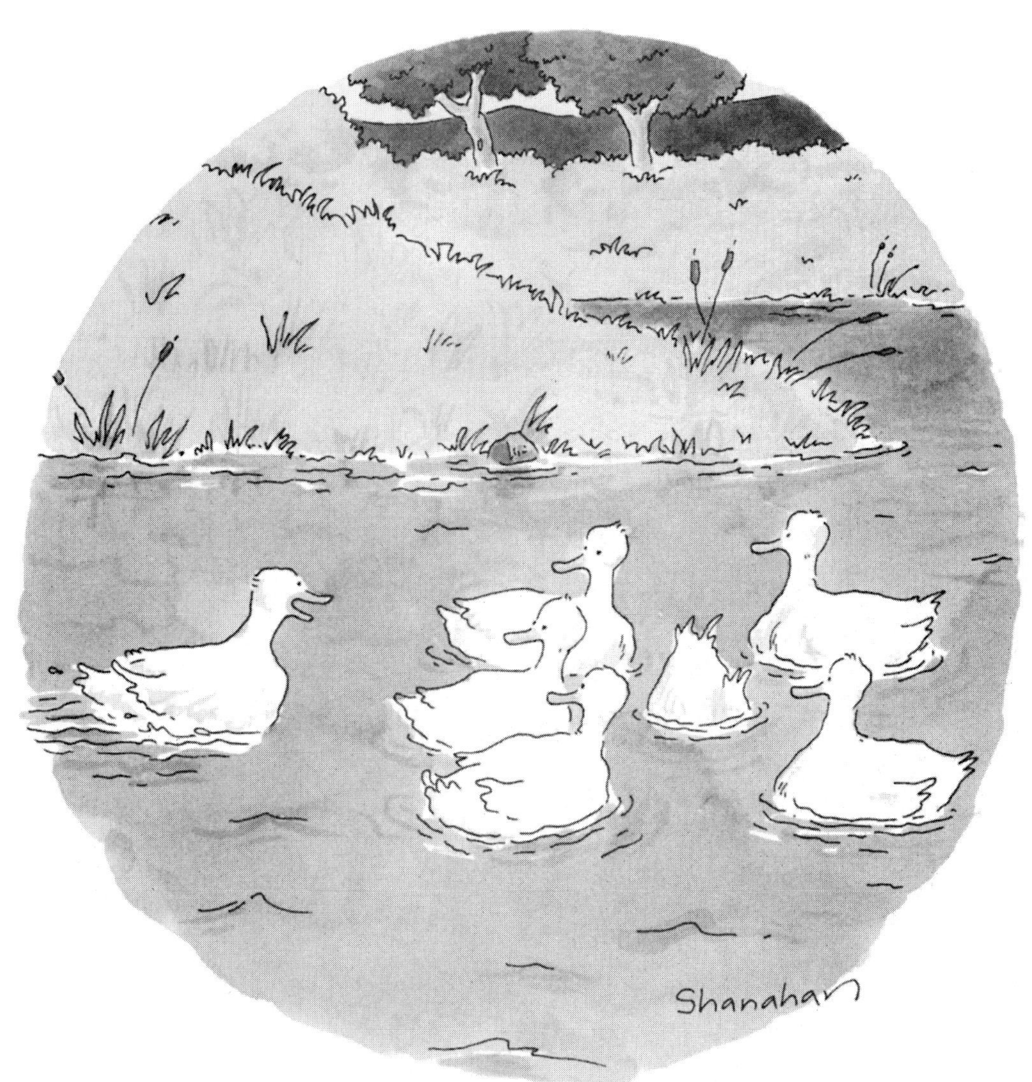

"Let me through! I'm a quack."

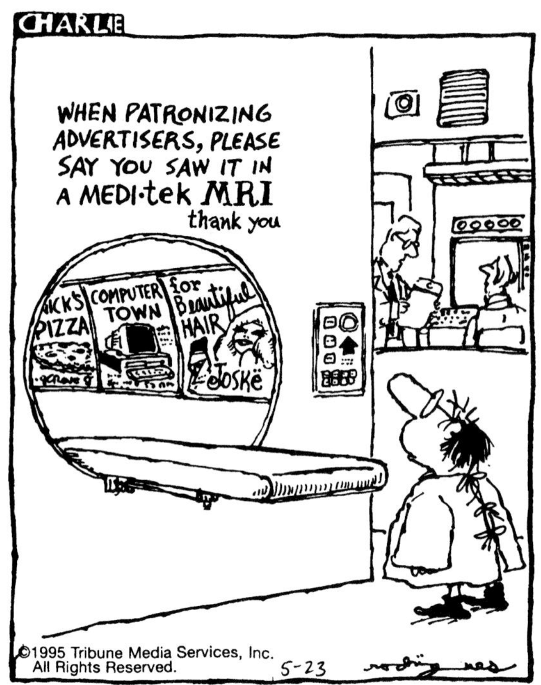

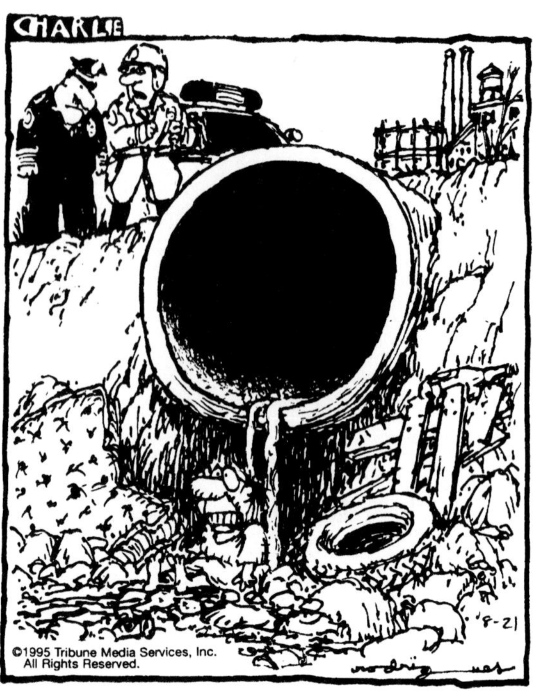

"All he knows, Sarge, is, five minutes ago he was placed in an MRI machine up on center street..."

Farcus

by David Waisglass
Gordon Coulthart

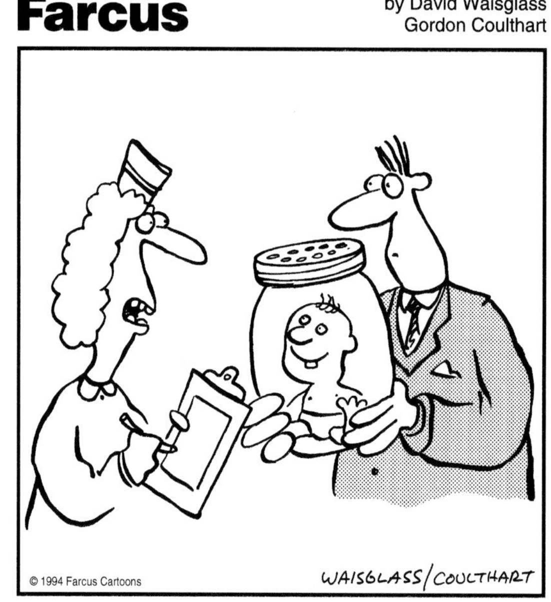

"I assume you're not the primary care giver."

Calvin and Hobbes

HEY, DOC, WHY ARE YOU RUBBING MY ARM WITH COTTON? ARE YOU GOING TO PUT A LEECH THERE?

ARE YOU GOING TO BLEED ME? YOU'RE NOT GOING TO AMPUTATE, ARE YOU? ARE YOU??

WHAT'S THAT? IS THAT A SHOT? ARE YOU GOING TO...
AAUGHH! IT WENT CLEAR THROUGH MY ARM!! OW OW OW OW!!!

I'M DYING! I HOPE YOU'VE PAID YOUR MALPRACTICE INSURANCE, YOU QUACK!!
WHERE'S MY MOM???
WATTERSON

SO DOCTOR, HOW IS YOUR GENE SPLICING RESEARCH GOING?
©1993 NORMAN DOG

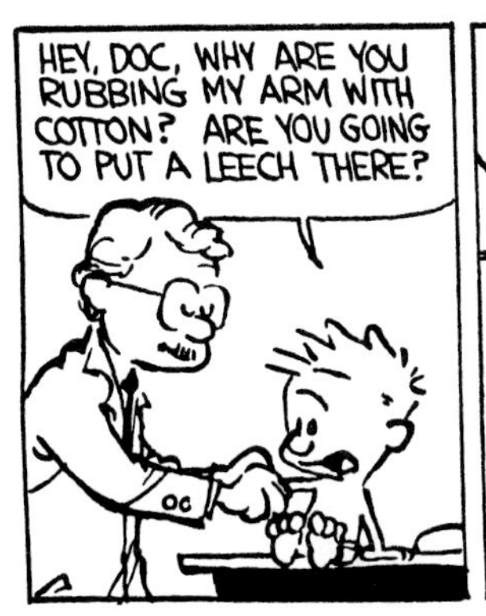

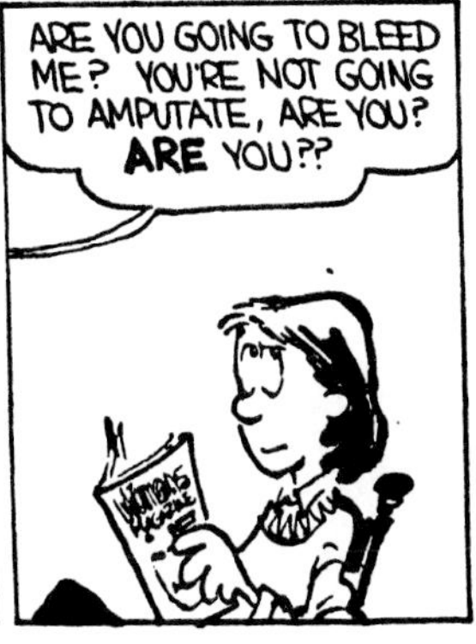

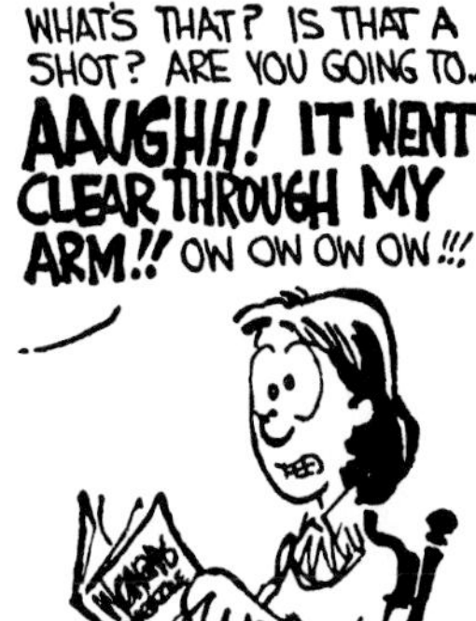

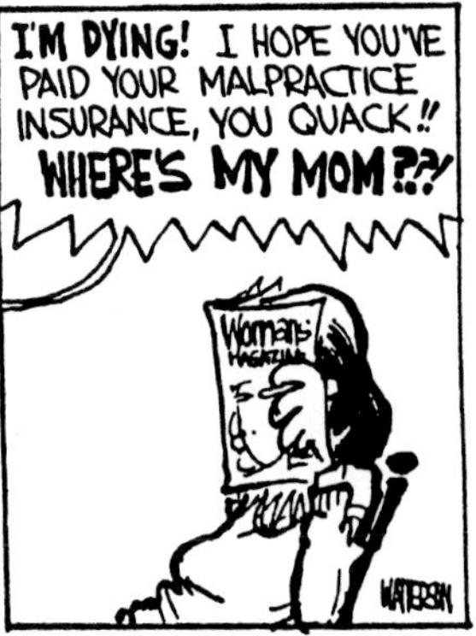

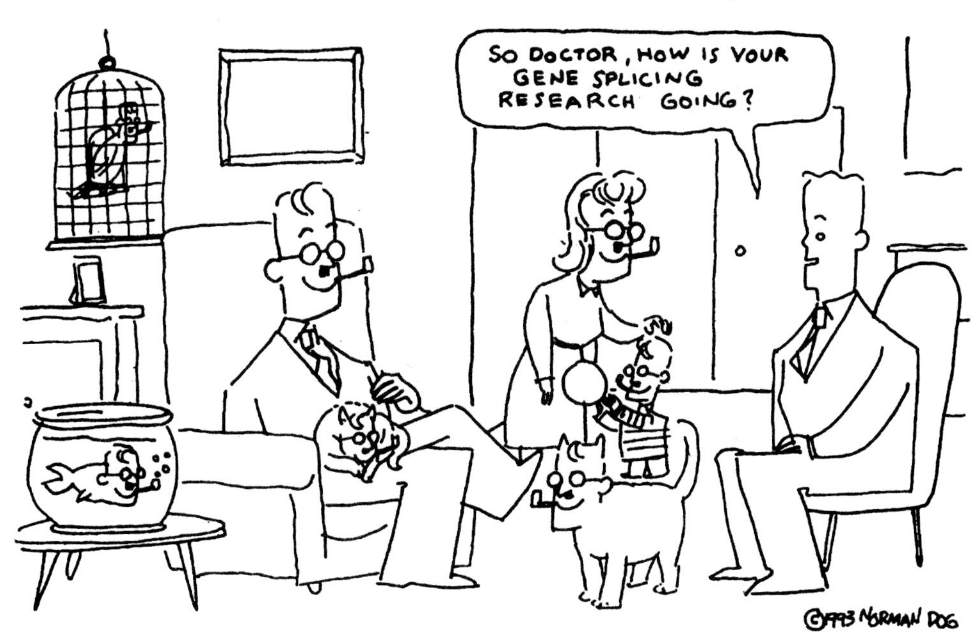

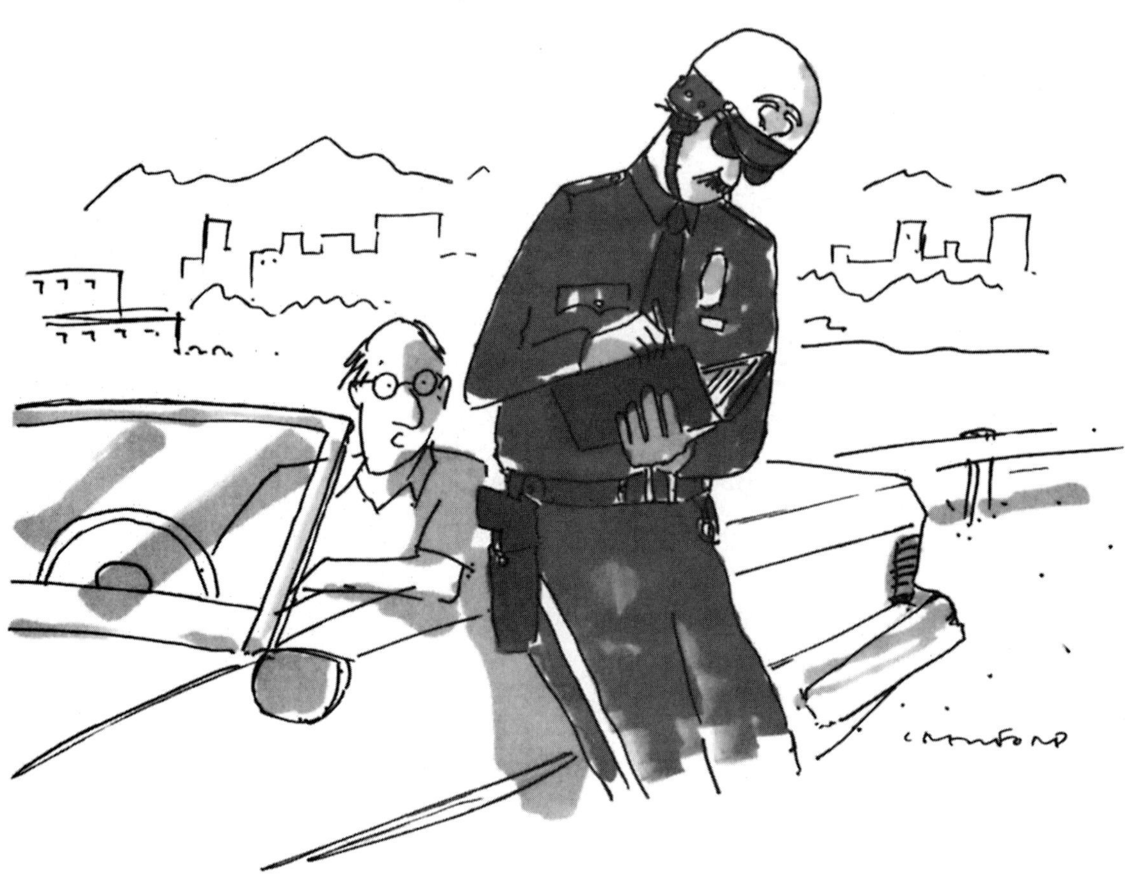

"Officer, shouldn't this be a time for healing?"

HERMAN®

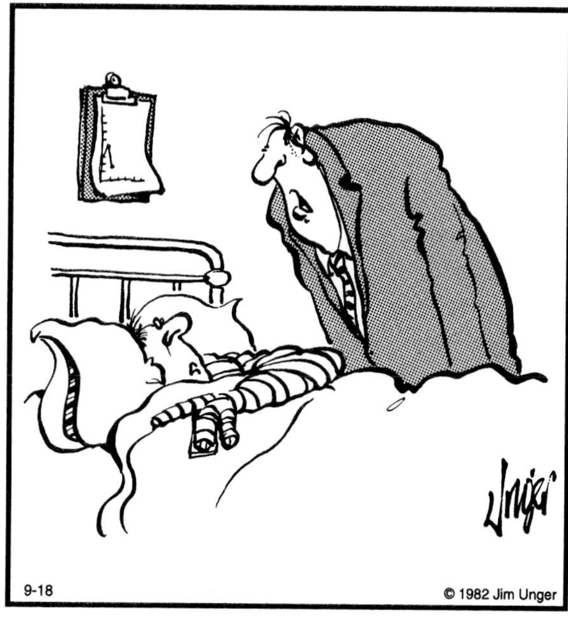

"I hate bothering you, but my wife wants to know if she passed her driver's test."

HERMAN®

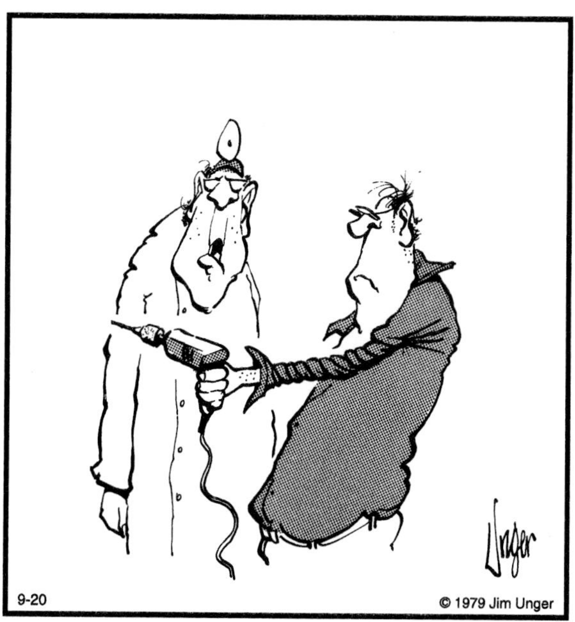

"Is there a reverse switch on the drill?"

HERMAN®

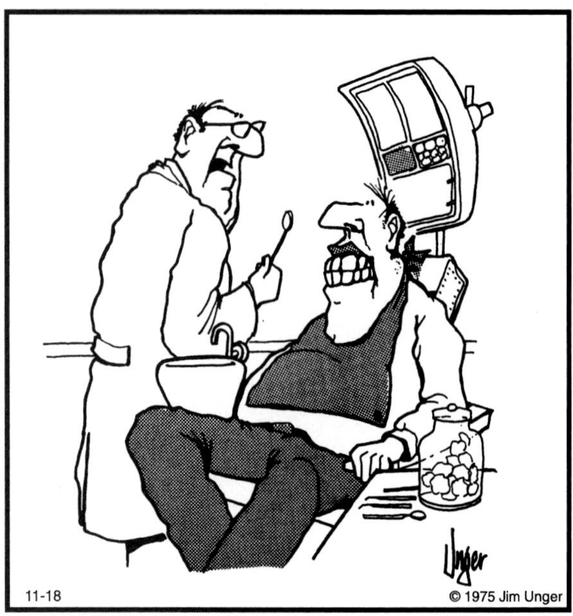

"It'll take you a couple of days to get used to them."

HERMAN®

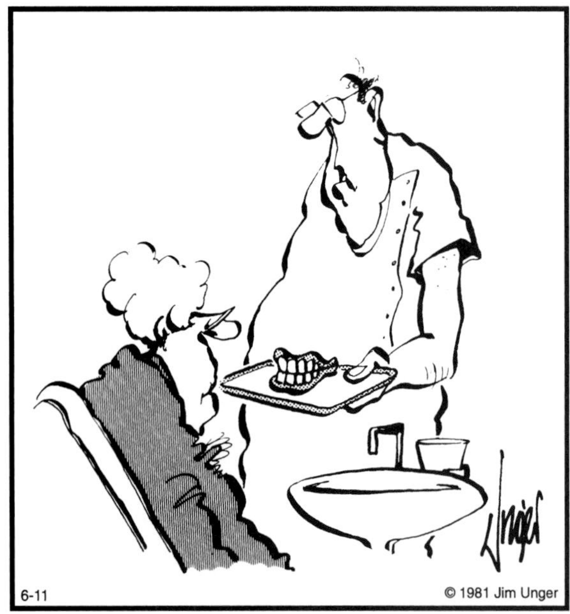

"These are expensive, but they're guaranteed up to 140 words per minute."

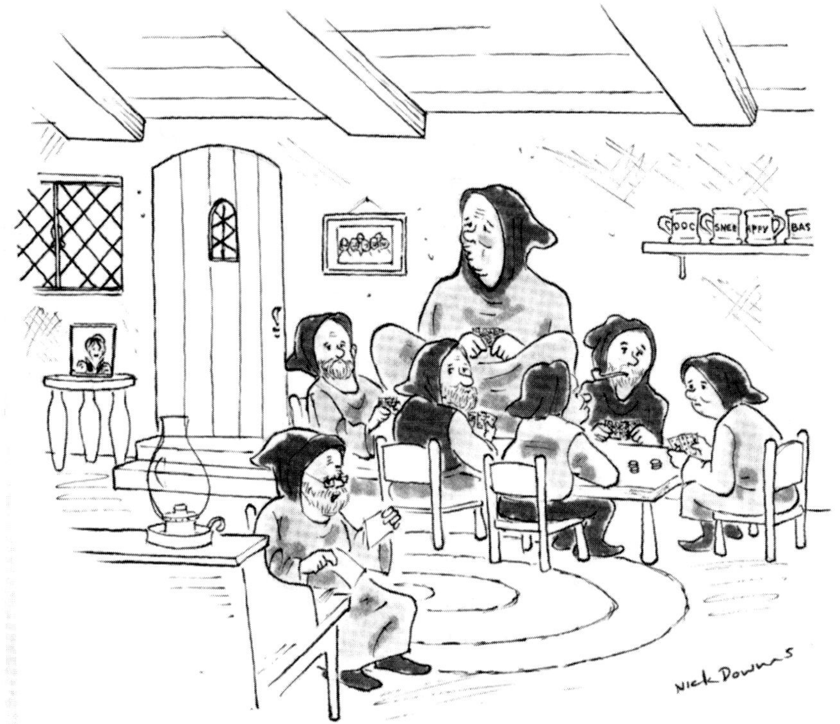

"What are all these bills from Genentech, Inc. ?"

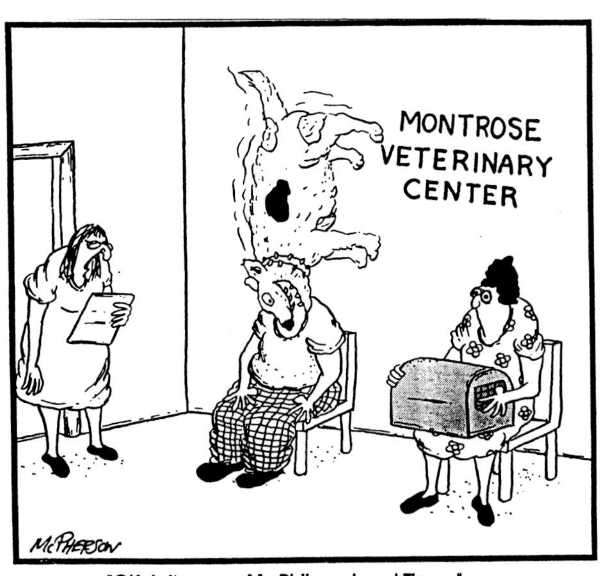

"OK, let's see ... Mr. Philmont and Tippy."

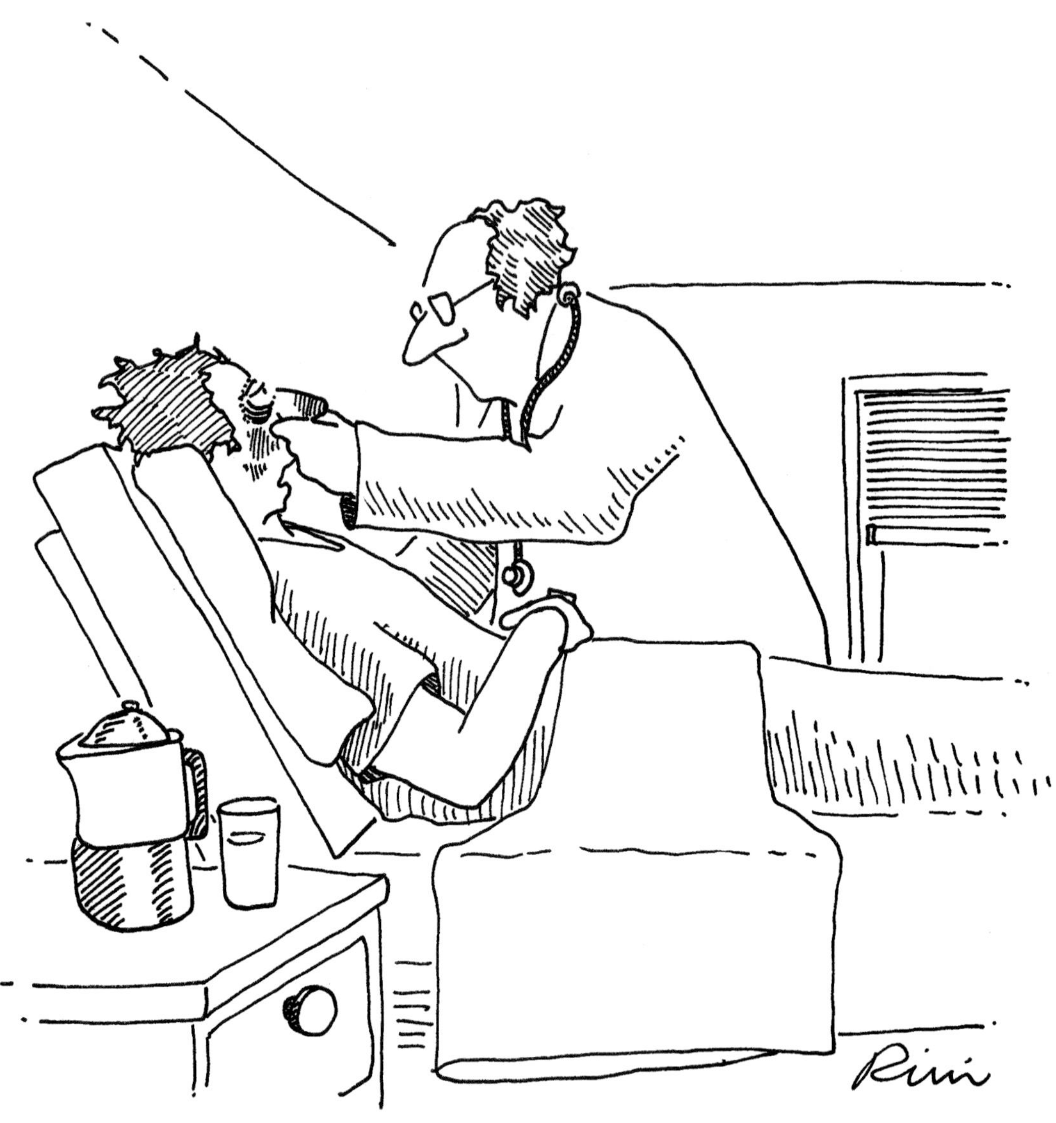

"**My life flashed before my eyes. Unfortunately, my wife was watching.**"

US & THEM by Wiley Miller & Susan Dewar

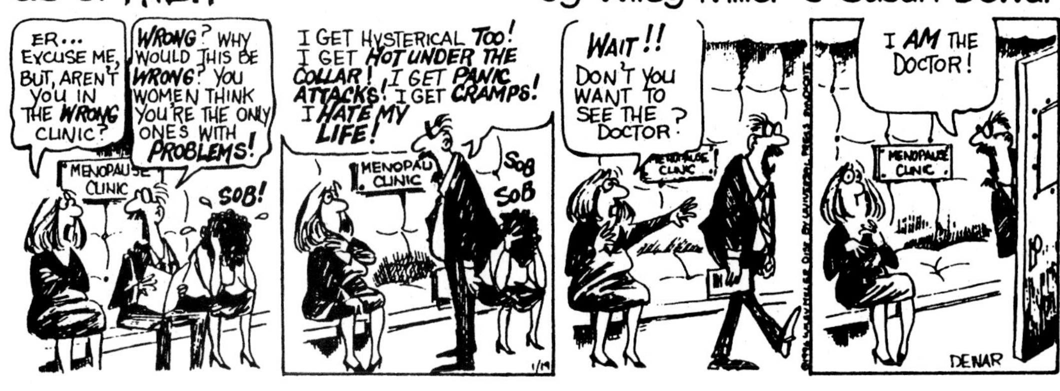

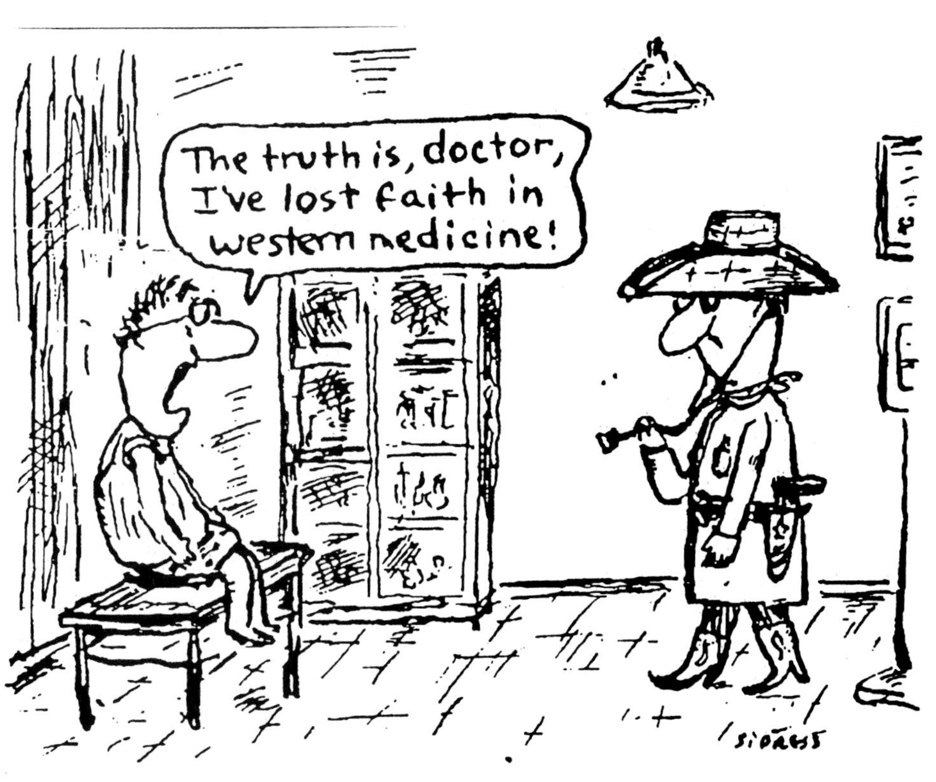

NEUROSURGERY
NEUROLOGY

"I need a song removed from my brain."

ALVIN KRONK, M.D.
EYE, EAR, NOSE,
AND THROAT.
LOUIS VARBER, M.D.
HEAD, SHOULDERS,
KNEES AND TOES,
KNEES AND TOES.

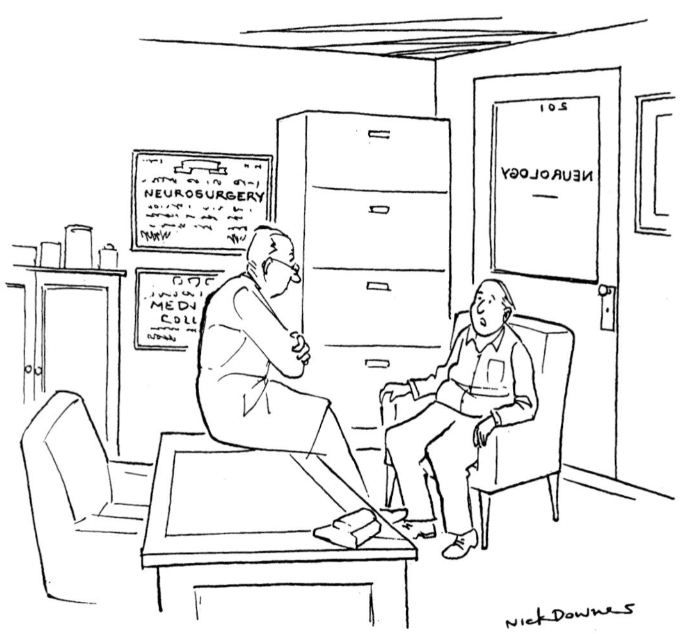

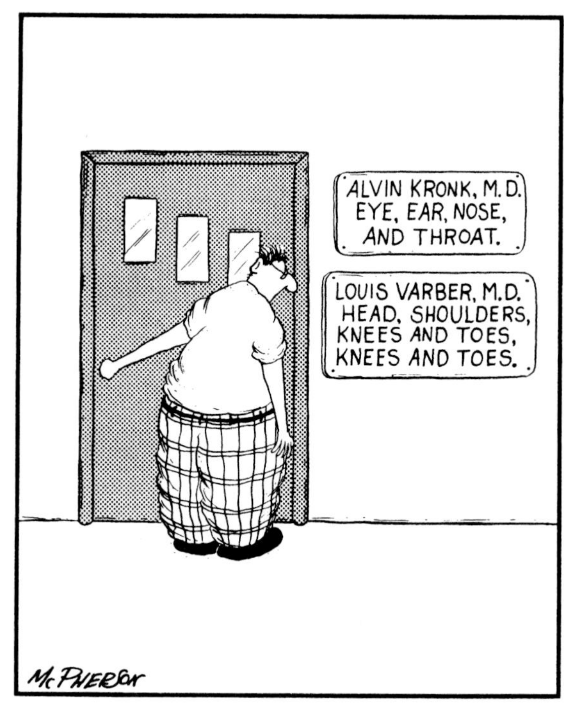

5.

Lifestyles of the Sick and Nameless

Smoked out

Dysfunction and dat function

Disorders of the highest order

It may feel good, but is it good for you

Good evening, and welcome to: "So You Think You've Got Problems?!!
SIPRESS

Callahan

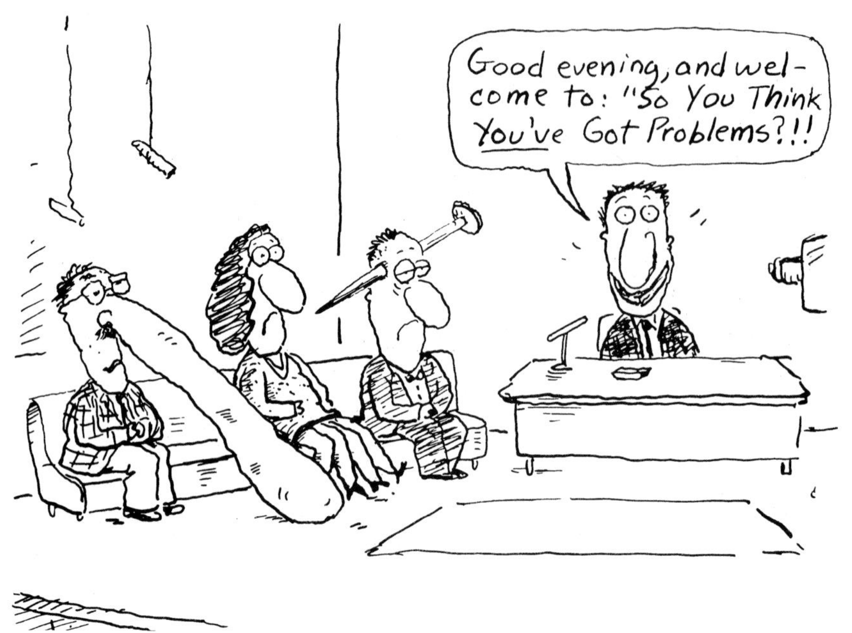

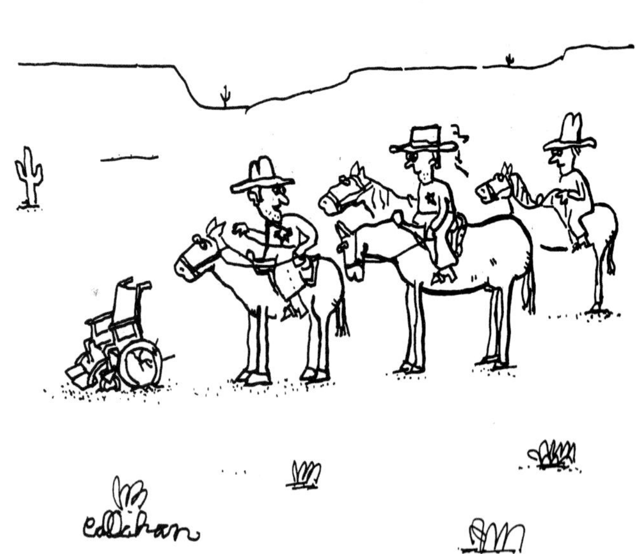

"Don't worry, he won't get far on foot."

THE FAR SIDE By GARY LARSON

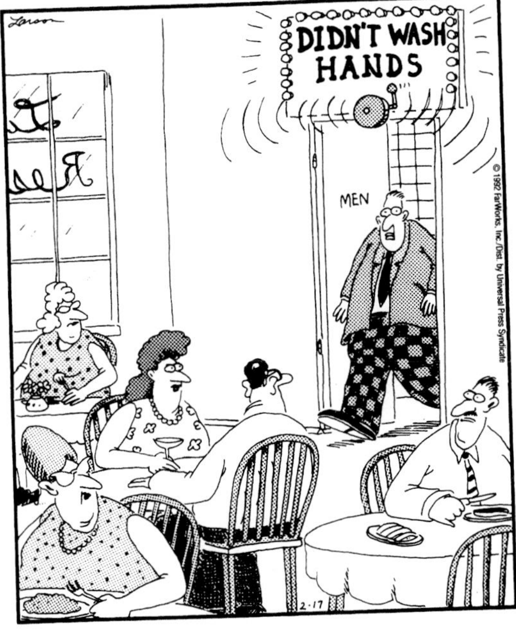

THE FAR SIDE By GARY LARSON

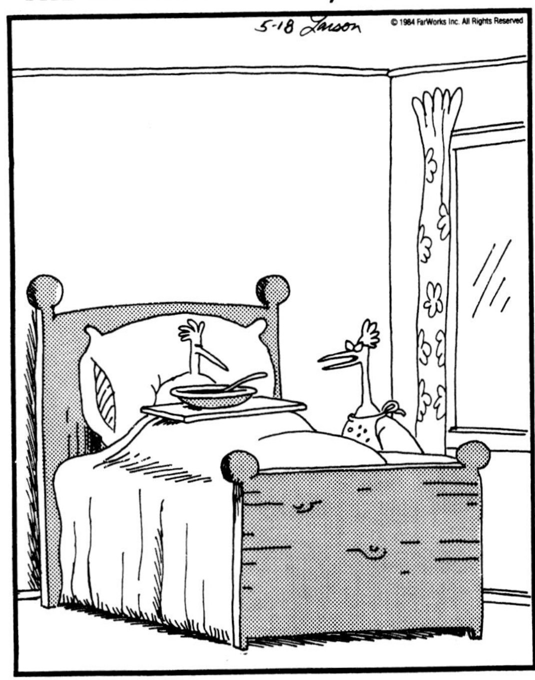

"Quit complaining and eat it! . . Number one, chicken soup is good for the flu — and number two, it's nobody we know."

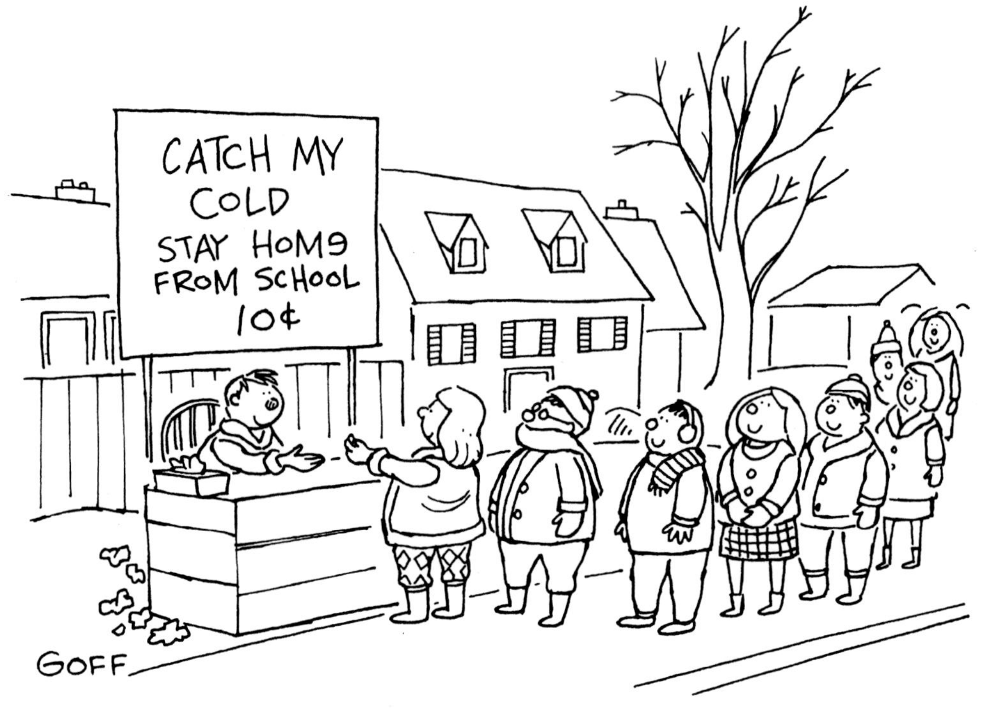
CATCH MY
COLD
STAY HOME
FROM SCHOOL
10¢
GOFF

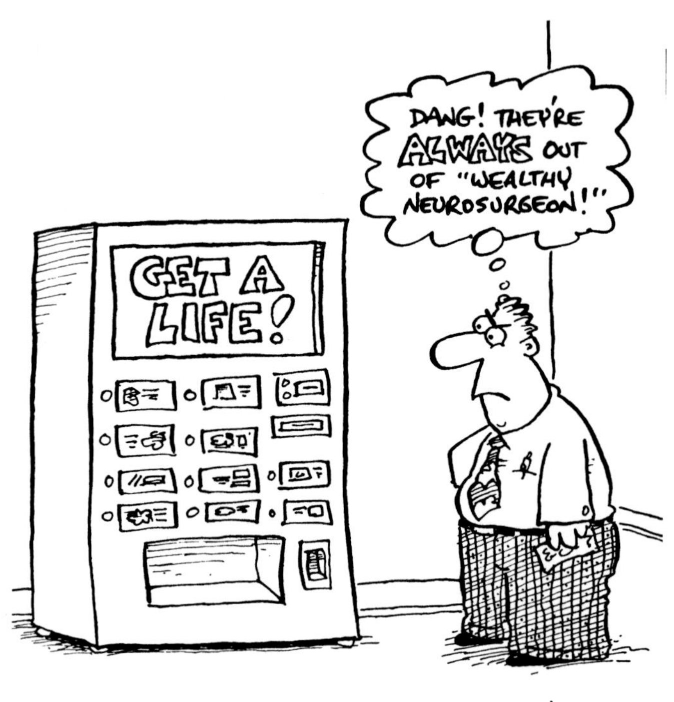
DANG! THEY'RE ALWAYS OUT OF "WEALTHY NEUROSURGEON!"
GET A LIFE!
VELEY

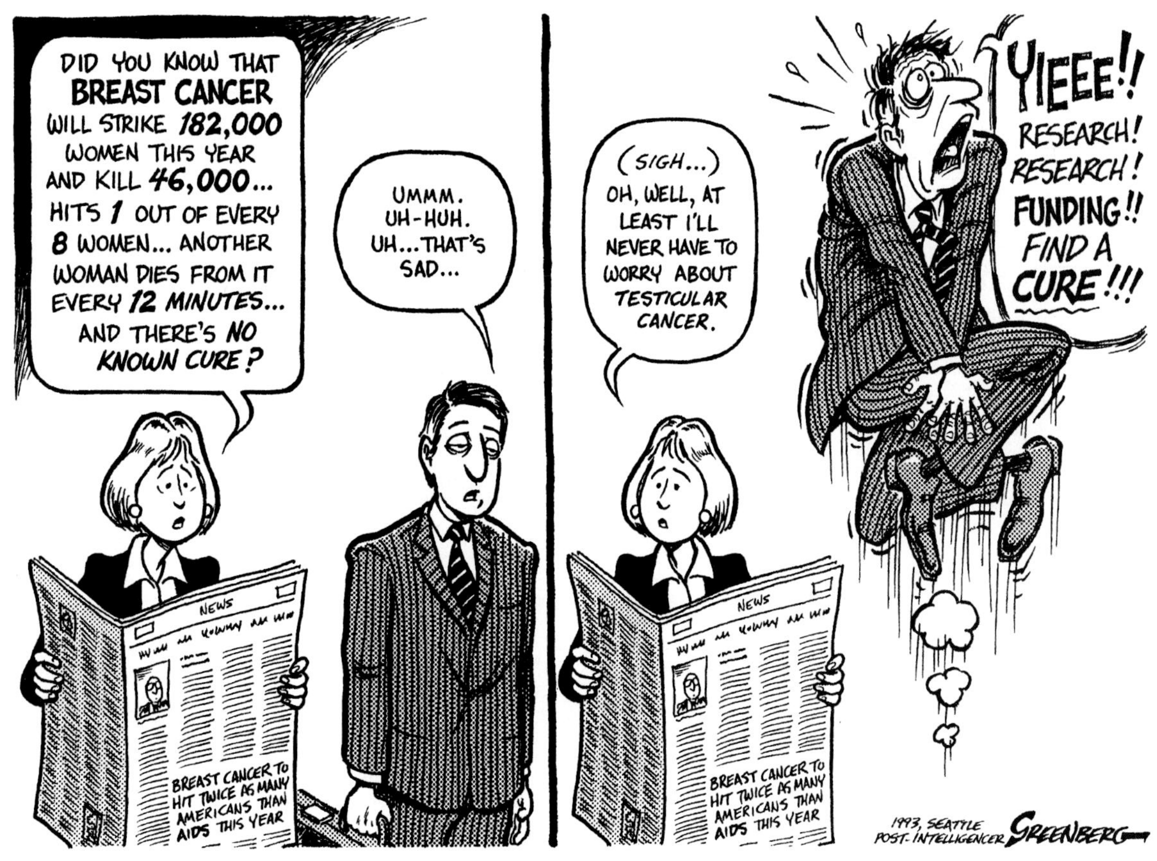
DID YOU KNOW THAT BREAST CANCER WILL STRIKE 182,000 WOMEN THIS YEAR AND KILL 46,000... HITS 1 OUT OF EVERY 8 WOMEN... ANOTHER WOMAN DIES FROM IT EVERY 12 MINUTES... AND THERE'S NO KNOWN CURE?
UMMM. UH-HUH. UH...THAT'S SAD...
NEWS
BREAST CANCER TO HIT TWICE AS MANY AMERICANS THAN AIDS THIS YEAR
(SIGH...) OH, WELL, AT LEAST I'LL NEVER HAVE TO WORRY ABOUT TESTICULAR CANCER.
NEWS
BREAST CANCER TO HIT TWICE AS MANY AMERICANS THAN AIDS THIS YEAR
YIEEE!! RESEARCH! RESEARCH! FUNDING!! FIND A CURE!!!
1993, SEATTLE POST-INTELLIGENCER GREENBERG

LIBBY REID/GIDEON BOSKER

Welcome to the chemotherapy support group.

HEY MR. INCONSIDERATE, I CAN LIVE WITHOUT YOUR SECOND HAND SMOKE!
McLAREN

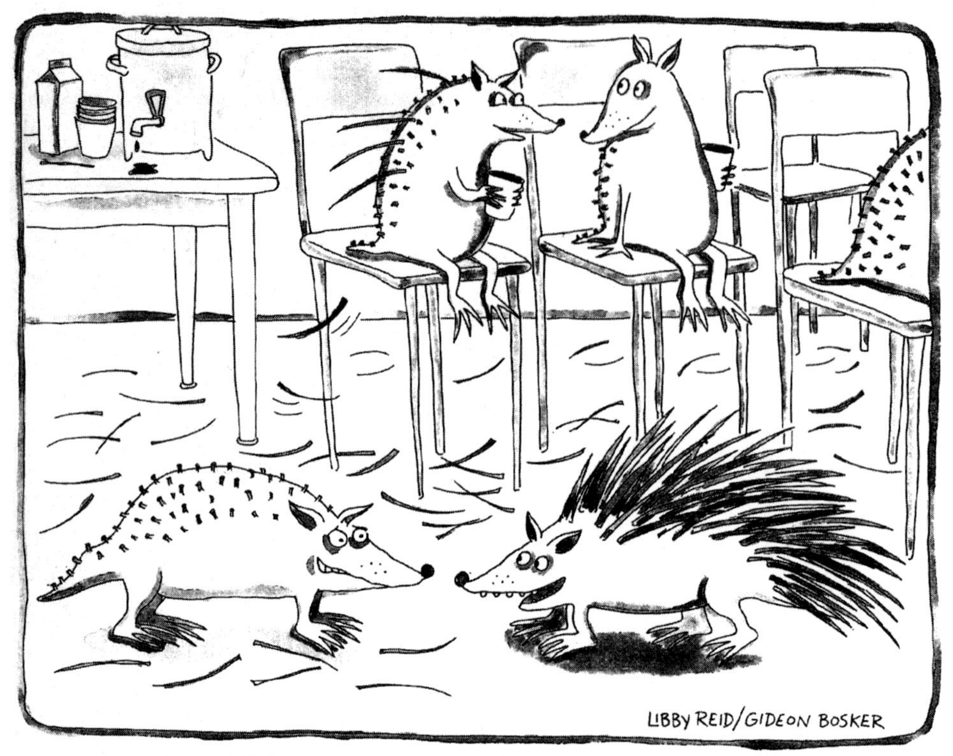

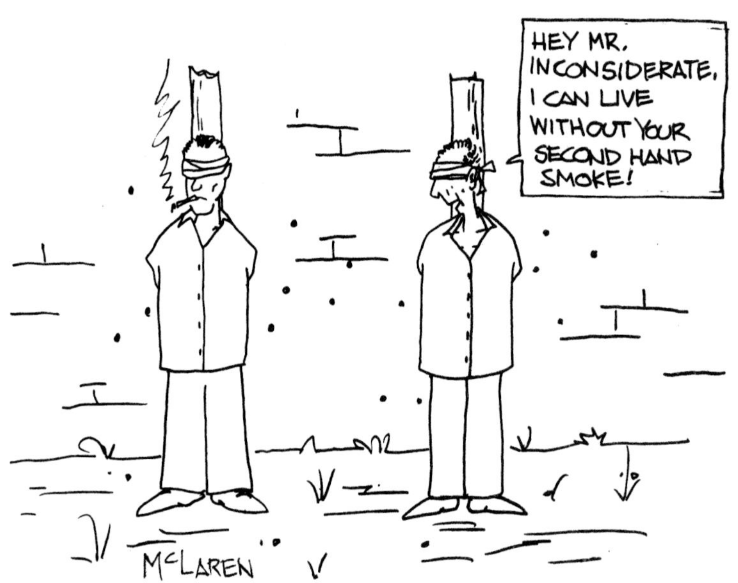

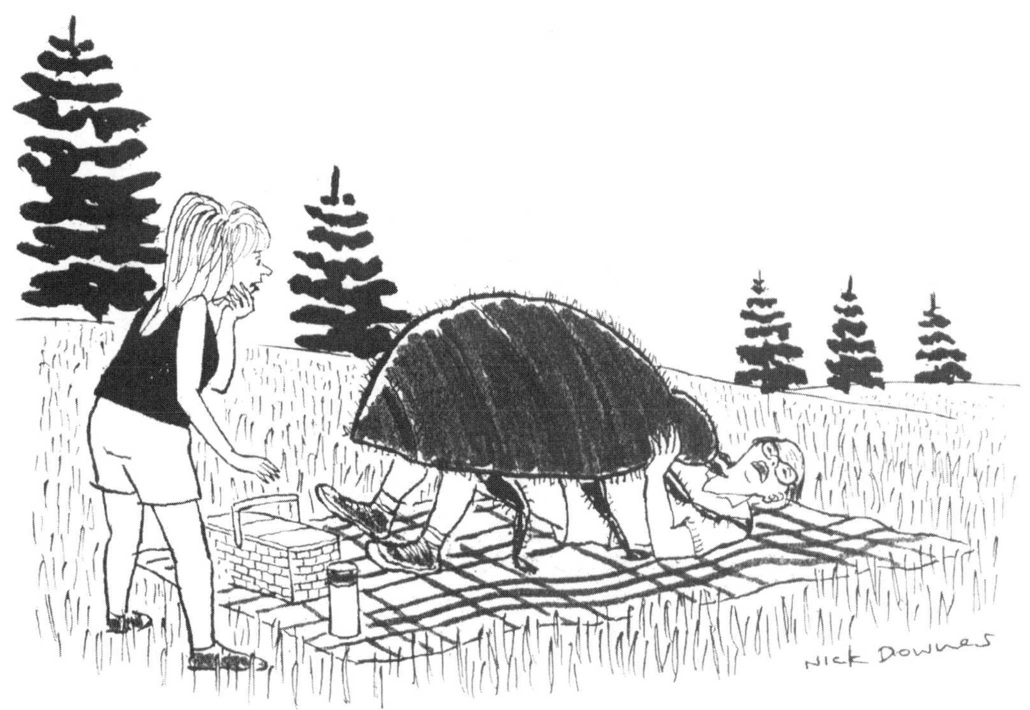

"First get him off me, Mary. Then we'll worry about Lyme disease."

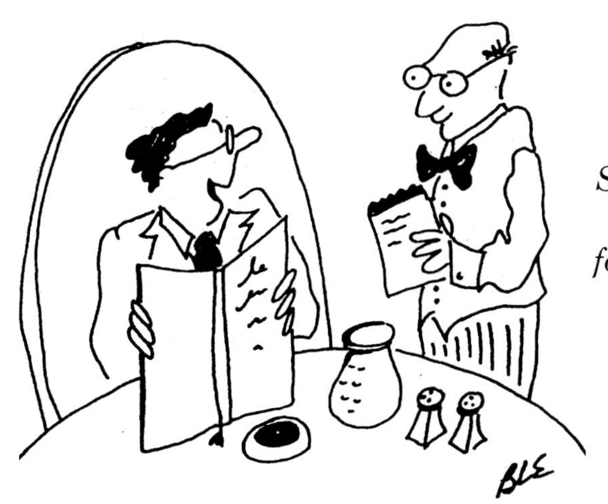

"I'll have the Cabernet Sauvignon for my cholesterol, the oysters on the half-shell for my cardiovascular system, and the French fries for my inner child."

HERMAN®

1-2
© 1987 Jim Unger

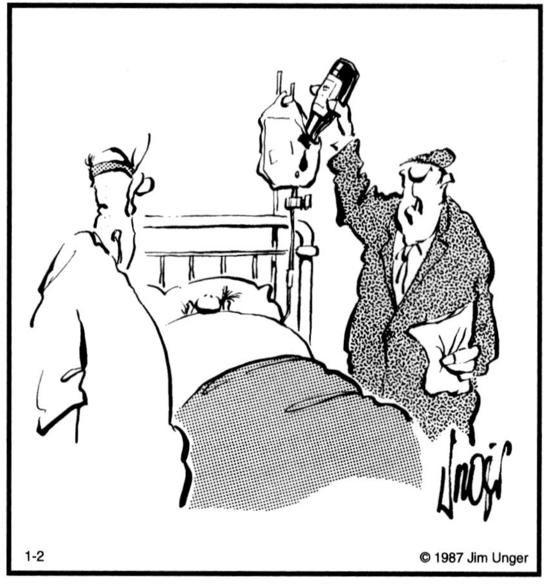

"He asked me to put some ketchup in here."

GEECH®

by Jerry Bittle

MR. BEEMER, DO YOU EXERCISE AT ALL?
RELIGIOUSLY.

MAINLY EASTER AND CHRISTMAS.

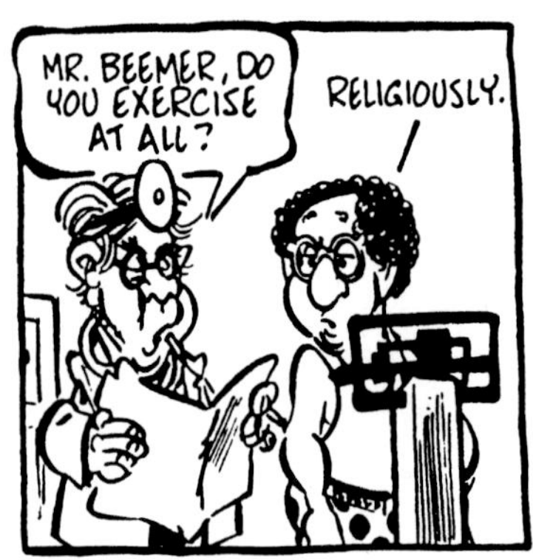

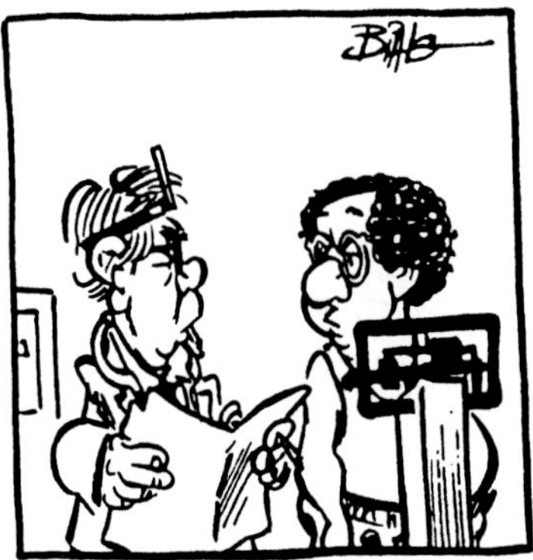

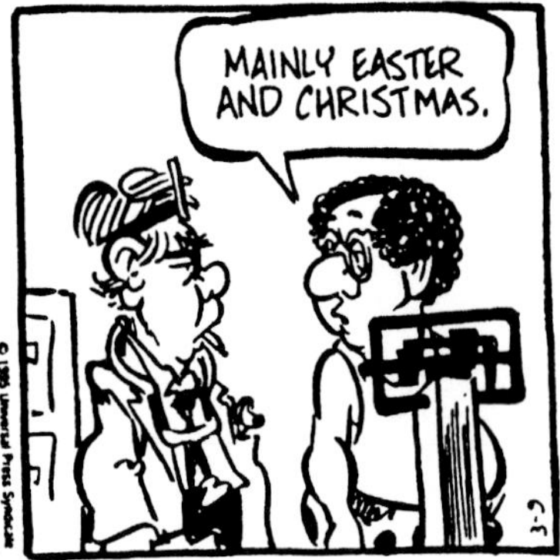

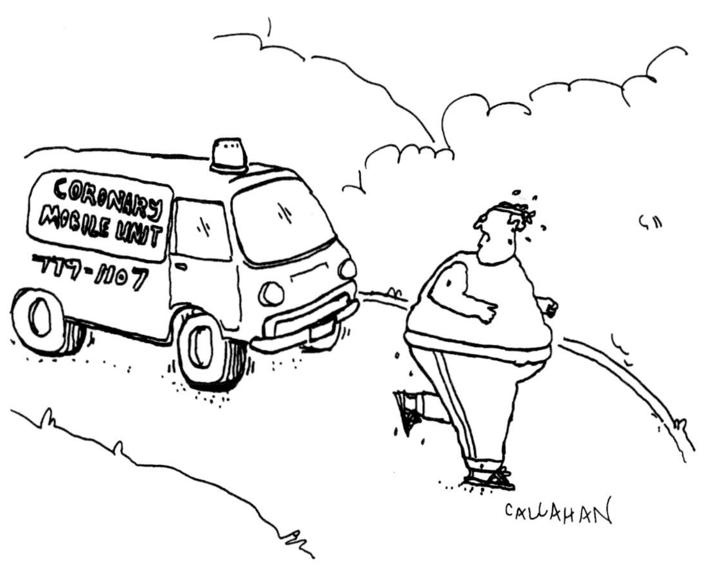

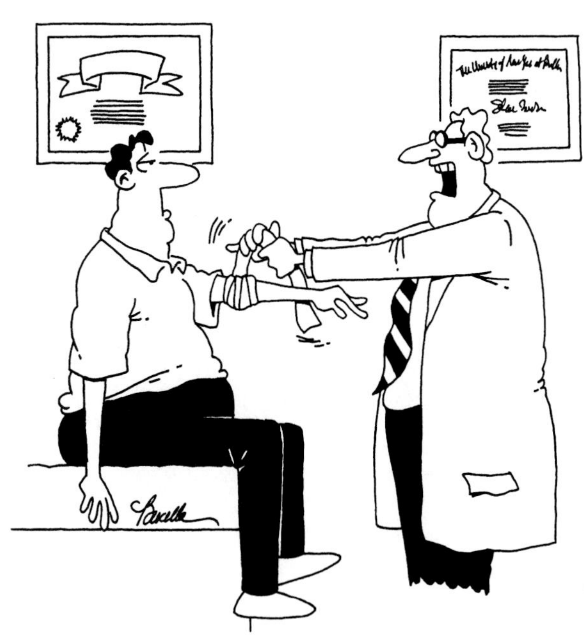

"Didn't anyone tell you that you're not supposed to light nicotine patches?"

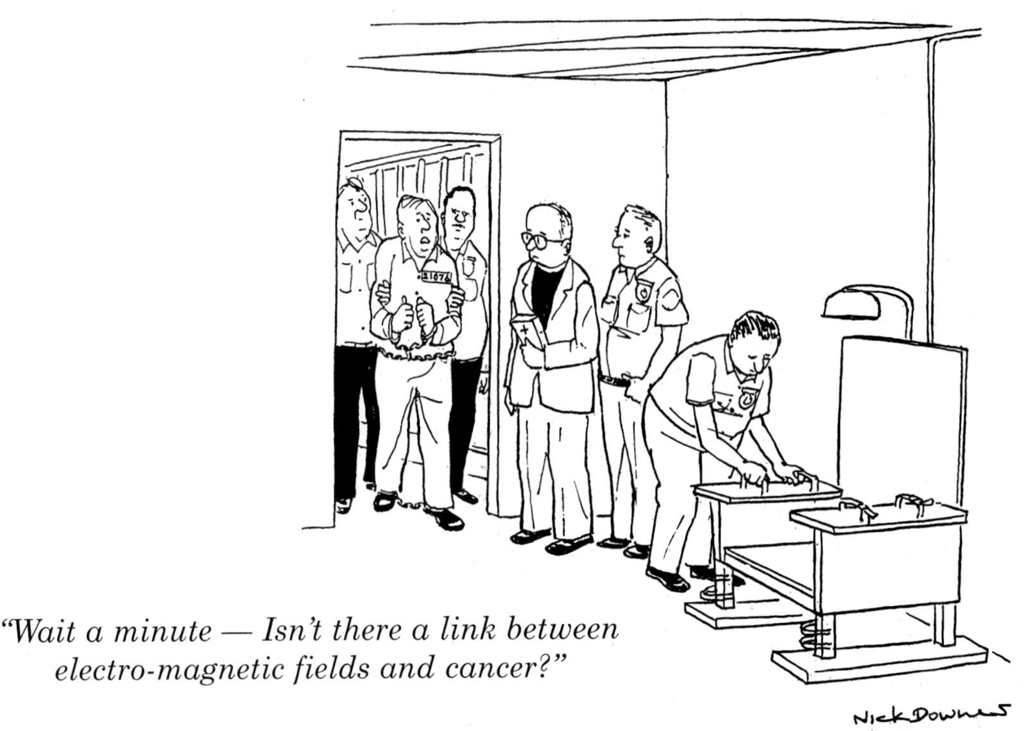

"Wait a minute — Isn't there a link between electro-magnetic fields and cancer?"

HERMAN®

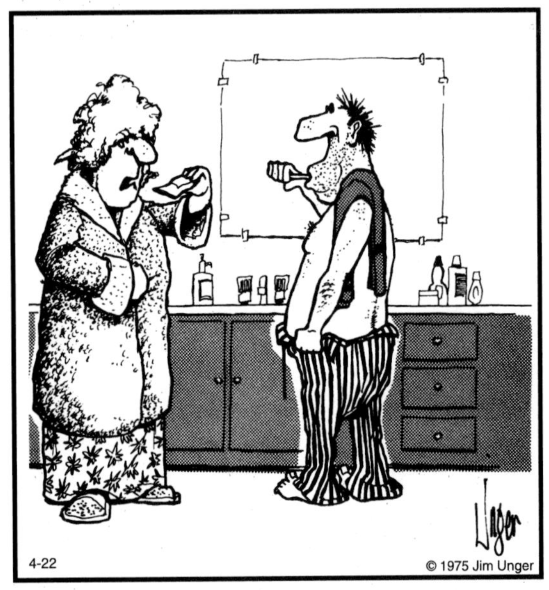

"You're using my athlete's foot ointment."

6.

Laugh Insurance

Managed care, Managed cost

Humorous Maintenance Organizations

Imagined Care Organizations

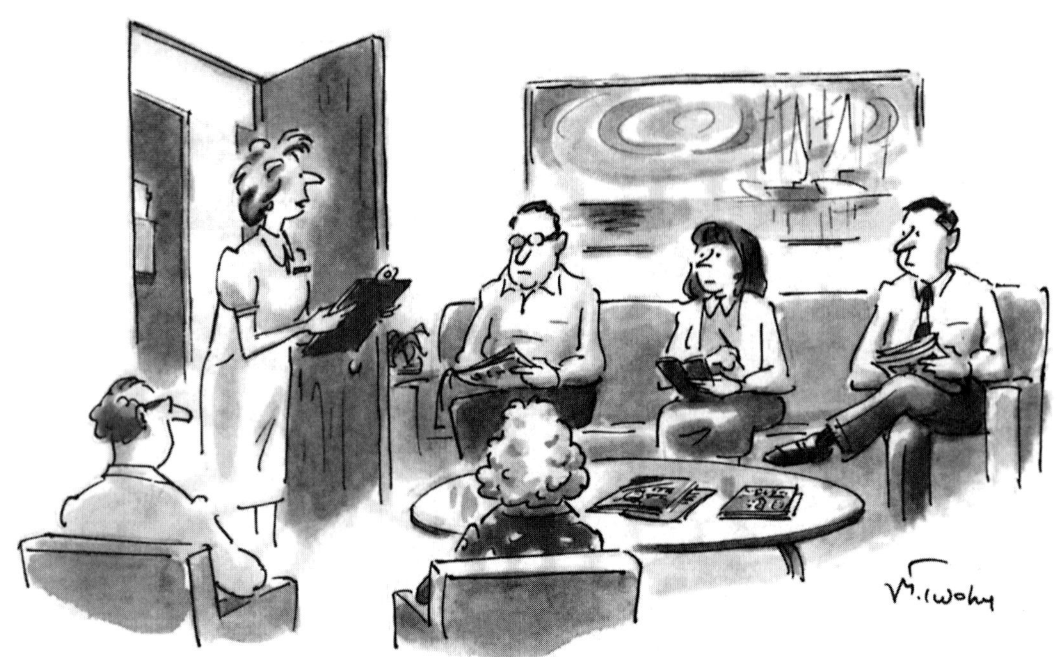

"Mr. Simpson, a doctor type will see you now."

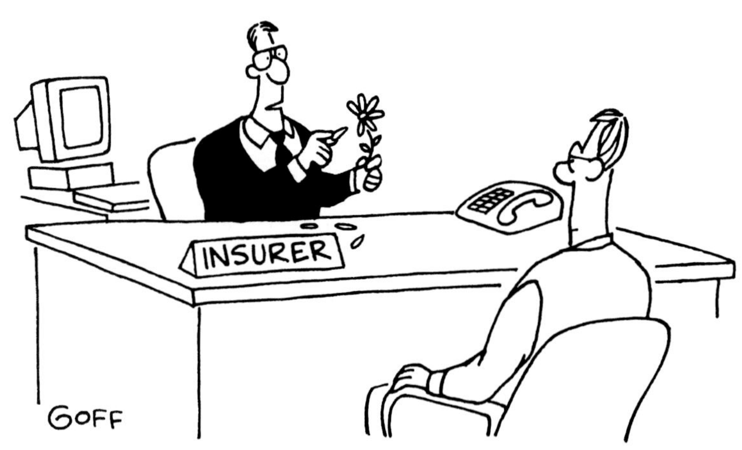

"WE PAY YOU, WE PAY YOU NOT. WE PAY YOU, WE PAY YOU NOT."

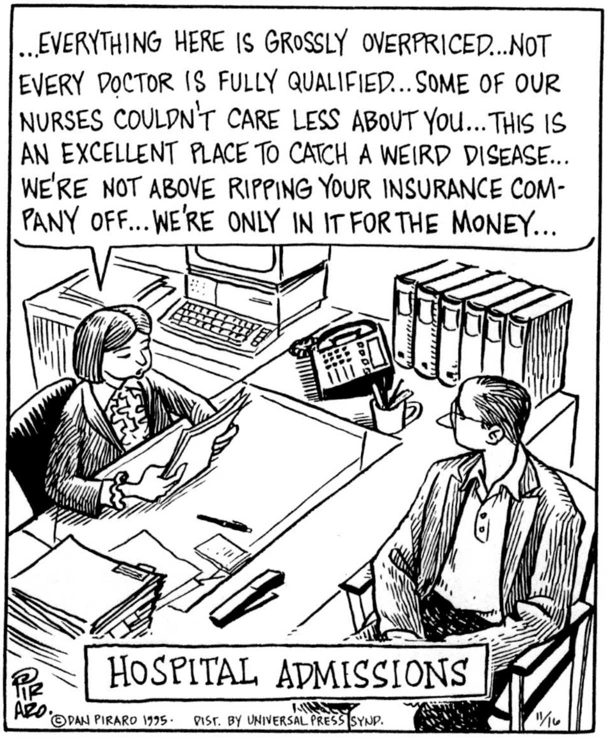

...EVERYTHING HERE IS GROSSLY OVERPRICED...NOT EVERY DOCTOR IS FULLY QUALIFIED...SOME OF OUR NURSES COULDN'T CARE LESS ABOUT YOU...THIS IS AN EXCELLENT PLACE TO CATCH A WEIRD DISEASE... WE'RE NOT ABOVE RIPPING YOUR INSURANCE COMPANY OFF...WE'RE ONLY IN IT FOR THE MONEY...

HOSPITAL ADMISSIONS

PIRARO.

11/16

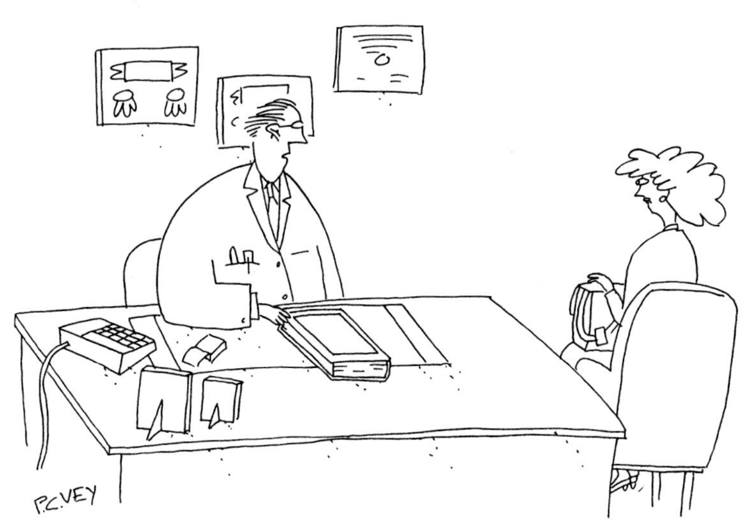

"I've taken the liberty of fictionalizing your test results. I hope you don't mind."

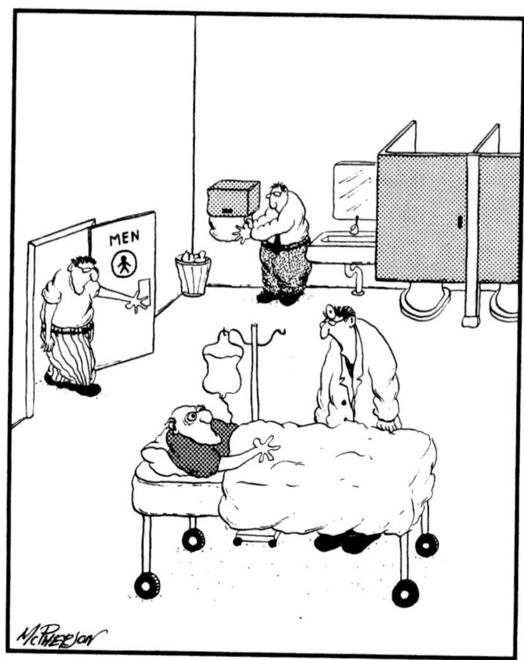

"Because, Mr. Westcott, your insurance doesn't cover the cost of a hospital room after gall bladder surgery."

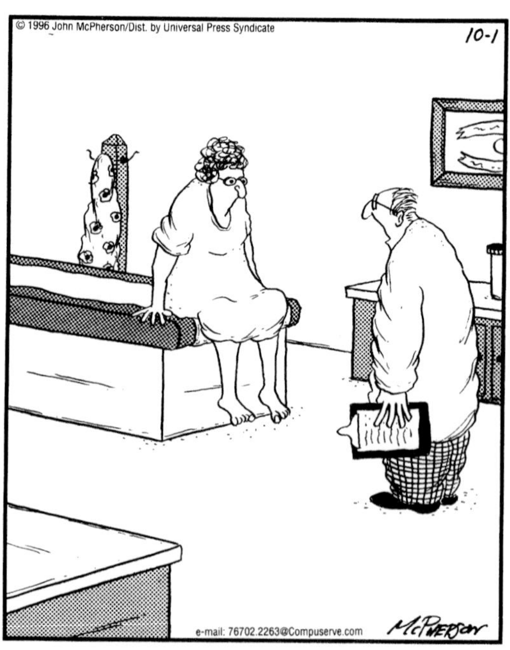

"I'm sorry, Mrs. Morris, but to prevent office visits from dragging on, the HMO requires that I answer only 'yes' or 'no' questions."

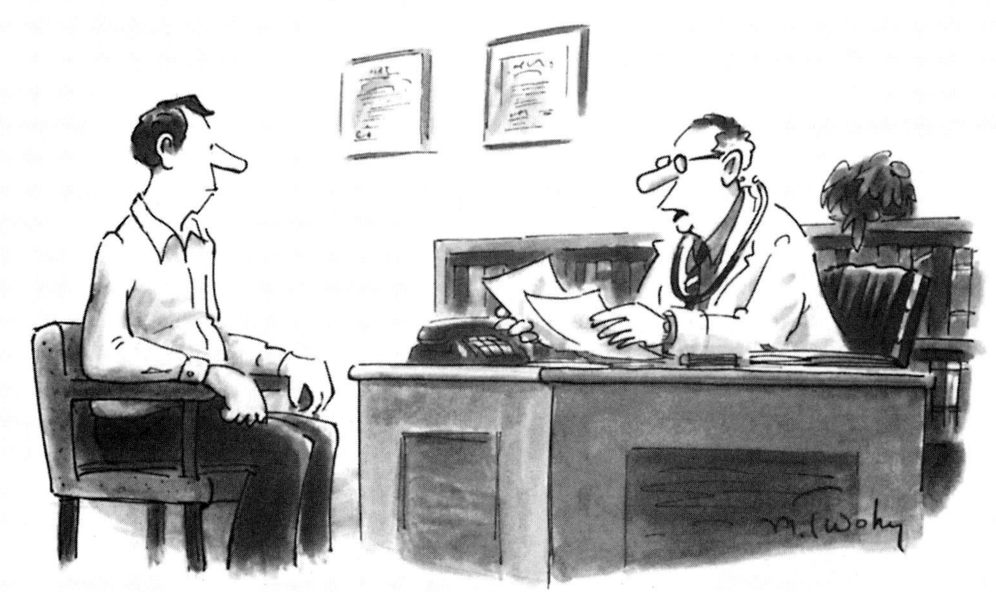

"I'll want to run a few tests on you, just to cover my ass."

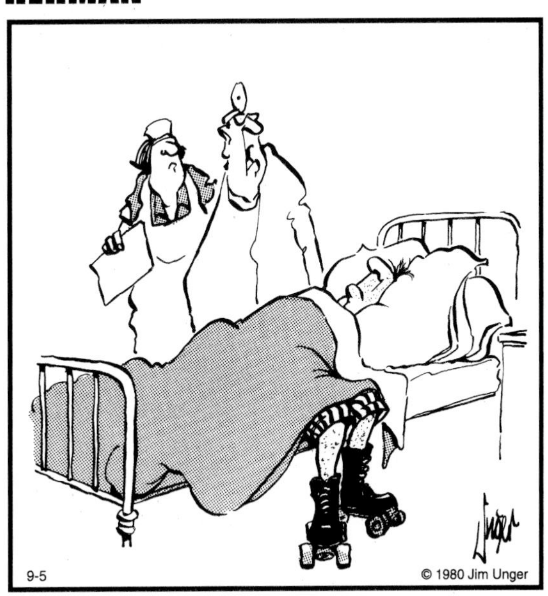

"Make sure this one doesn't leave before he pays his bill."

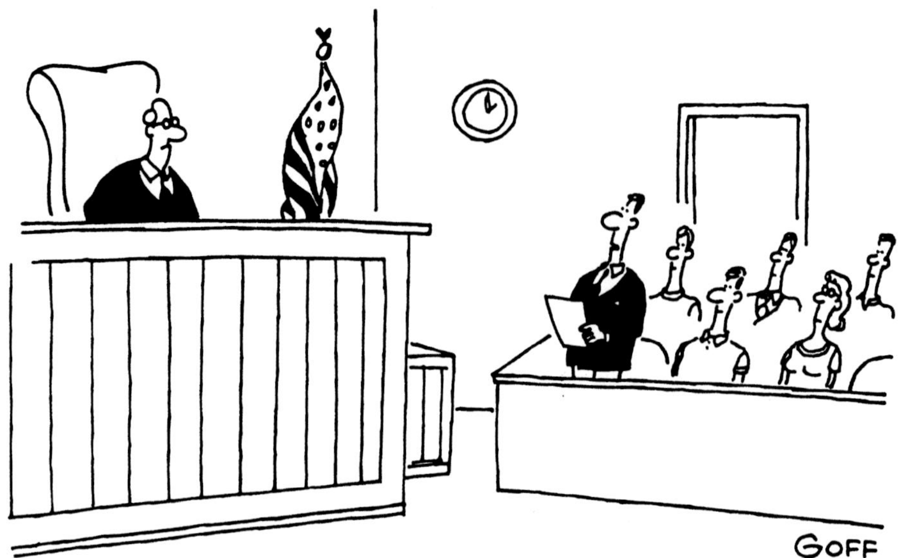

"Your honor, before we settle on a judgment amount, we'd like to know how much money there is in the universe."

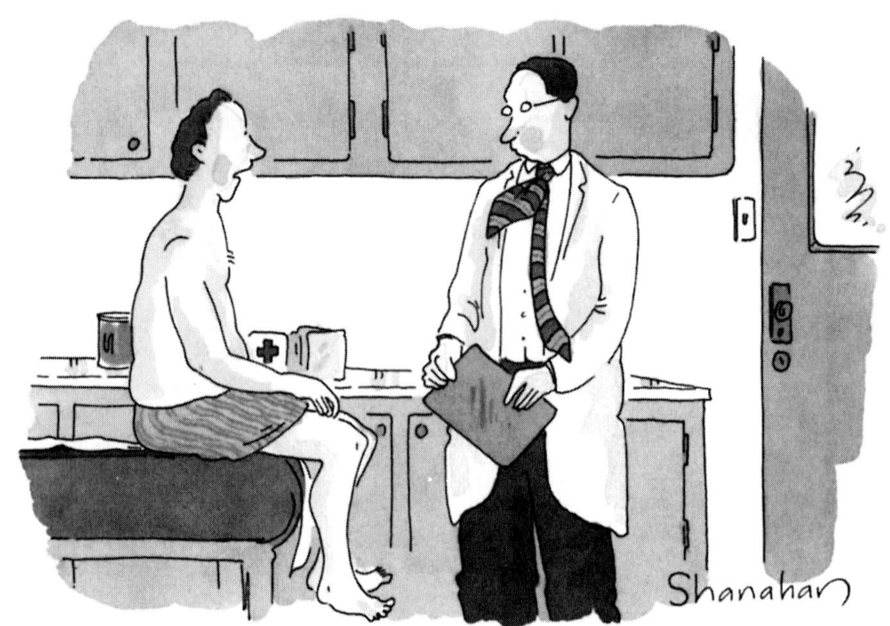

"And would you be performing the actual surgery?"

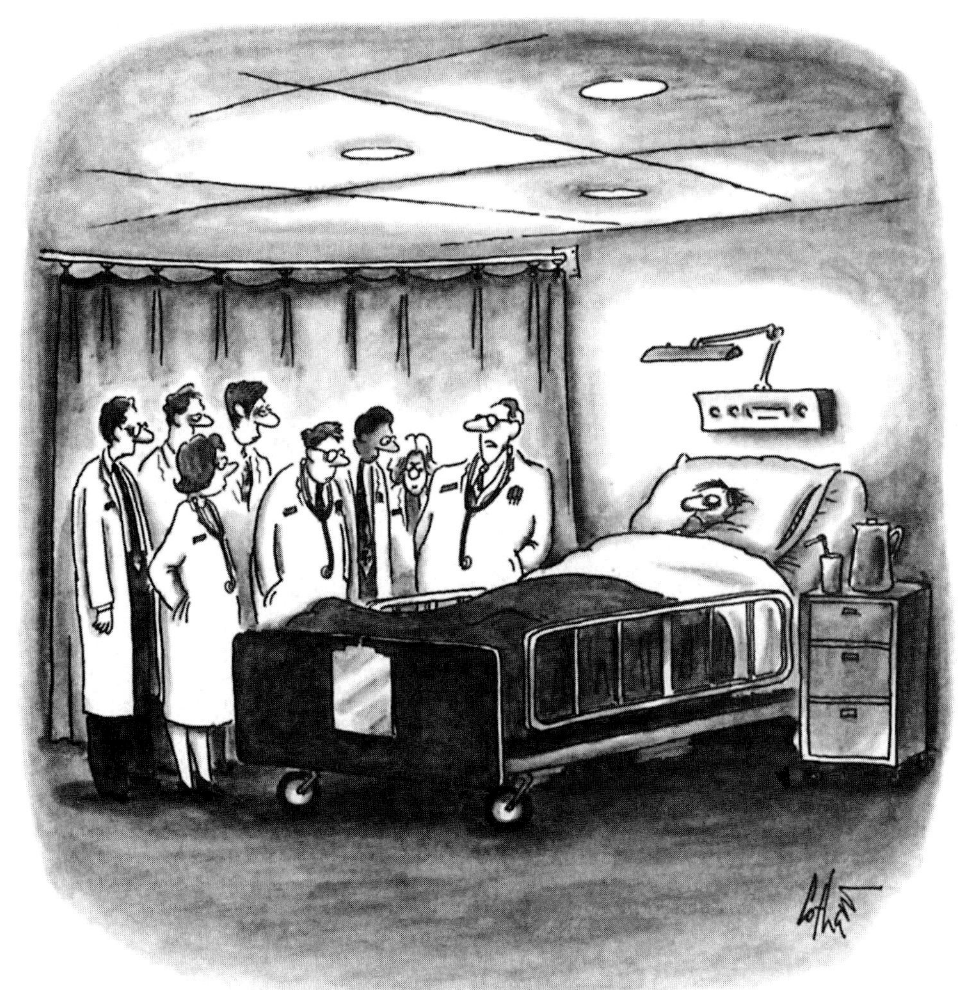

"This patient has a rare form of medical insurance."

BUT JOSEPH. WHY MUST WE TRAVEL TO BETHLEHEM?
THATS THE LOCATION OF OUR PRIMARY CARE HMO PROVIDER...

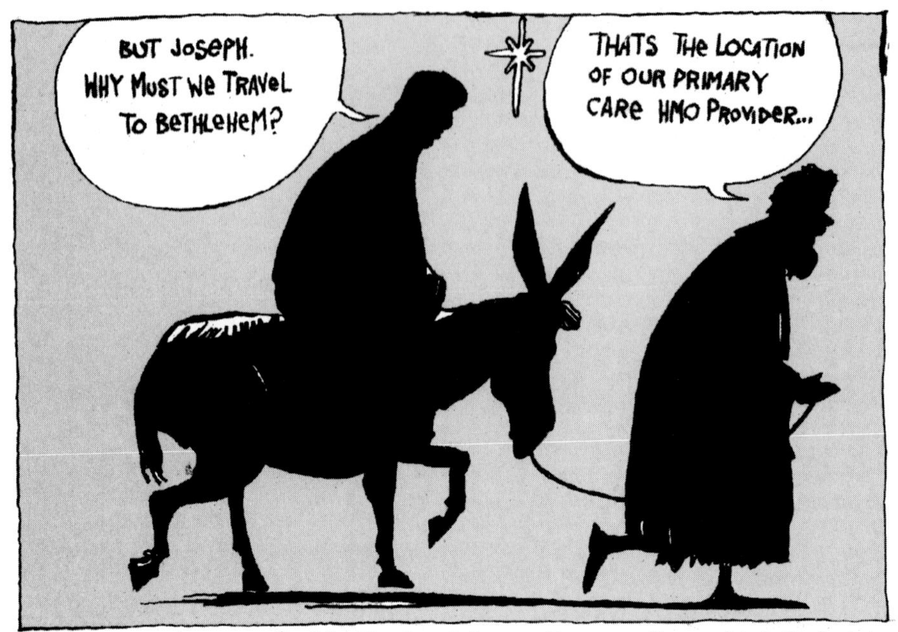

By John Deering, Arkansas Democrat-Gazett, Little Rock, Ark.

Farcus
by David Waisglass
Gordon Coulthart
© 1993 Farcus Cartoons
WAISGLASS/COULTHART

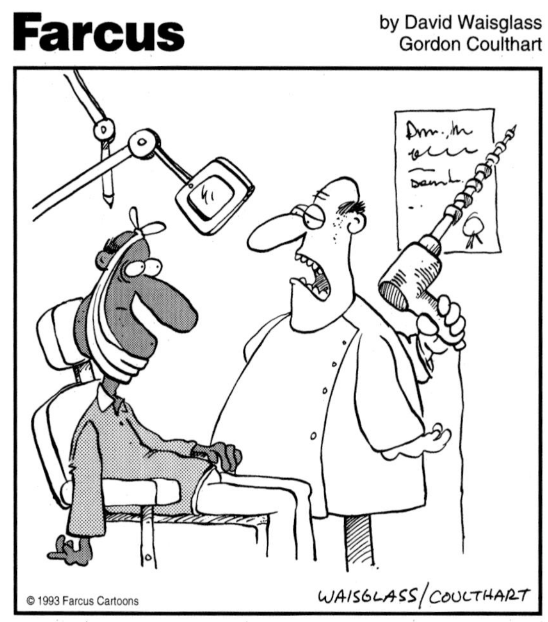

**"There are two ways to do this ...
Do you have a dental plan?"**

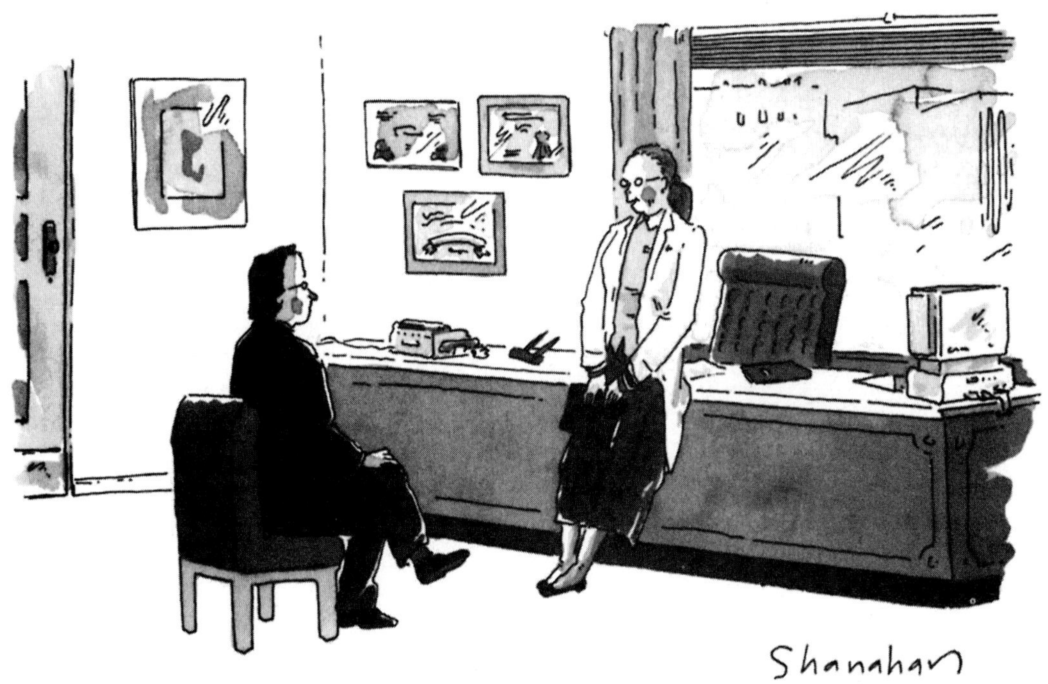

"Our integrated approach to medicine skillfully combines an array of holistic alternative treatments with a sophisticated computerized billing service."

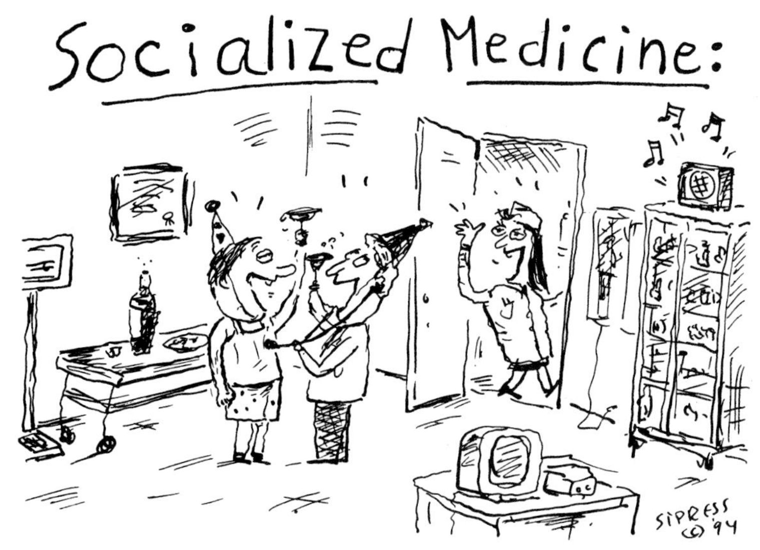

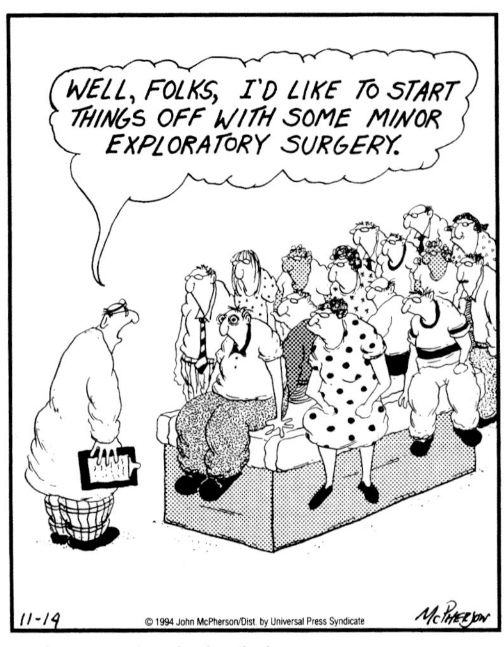

Gary was beginning to have some concerns about his new group health plan.

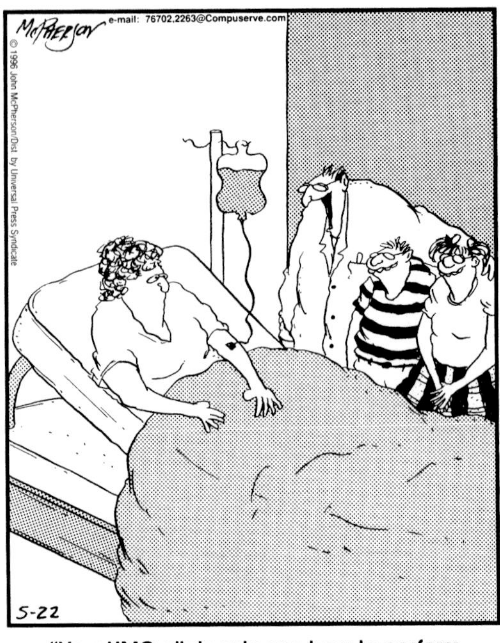

"Your HMO allots only one hour to perform hip-replacement surgery. After that, our candy stripers Chip and Brenda will take over."

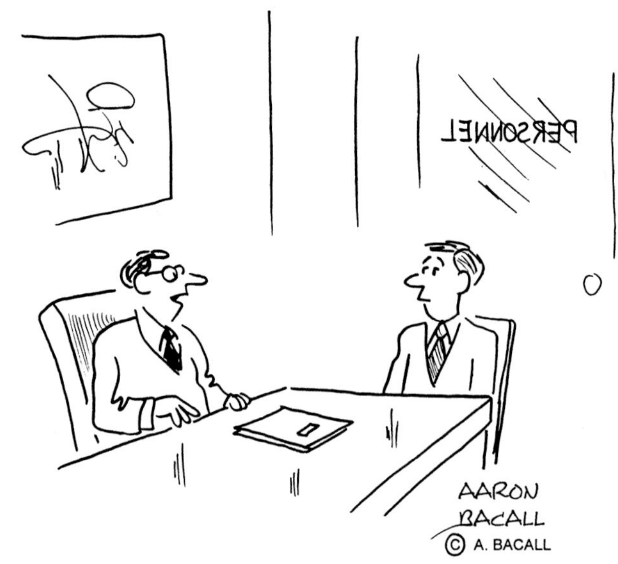

"We offer excellent medical coverage but the policy does not cover pre-existing organs."

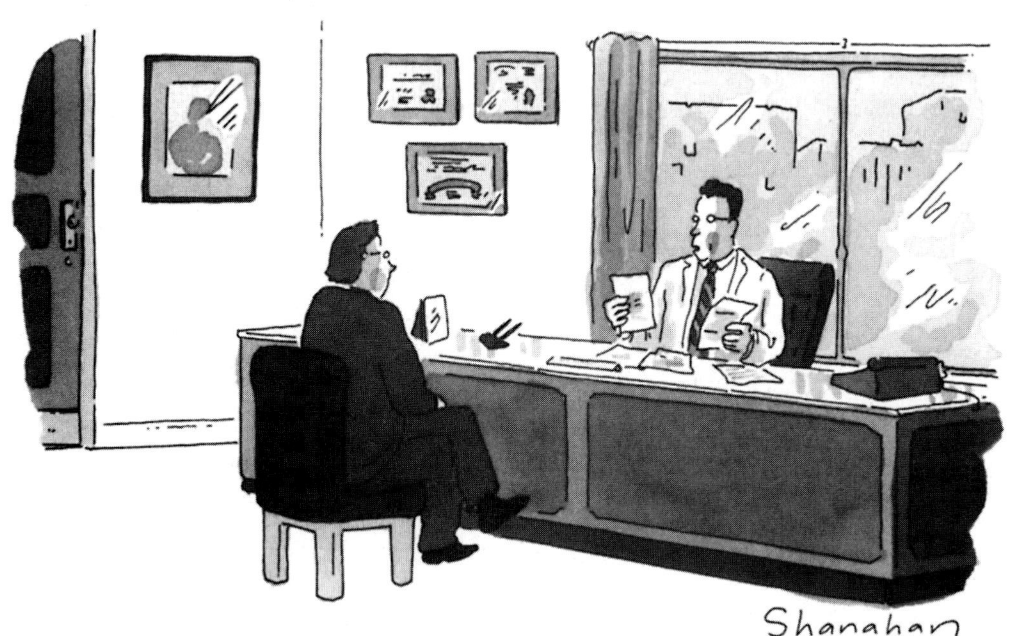

"You're responding beautifully. Let's go ahead and see what happens if we increase your deductible."

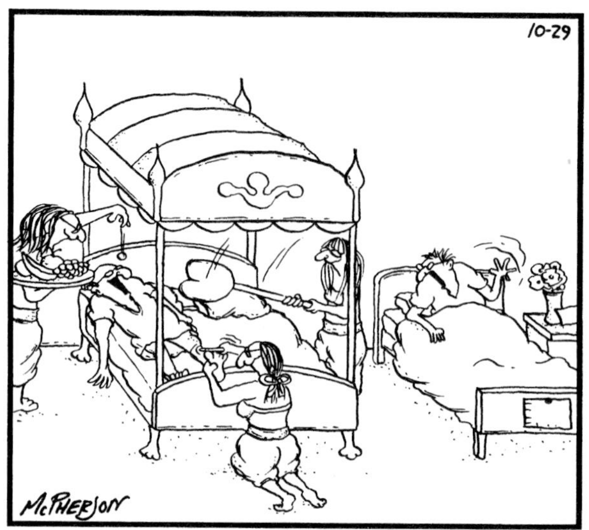

"For cryin' out loud! What the heck kind of health insurance do you have anyway?"

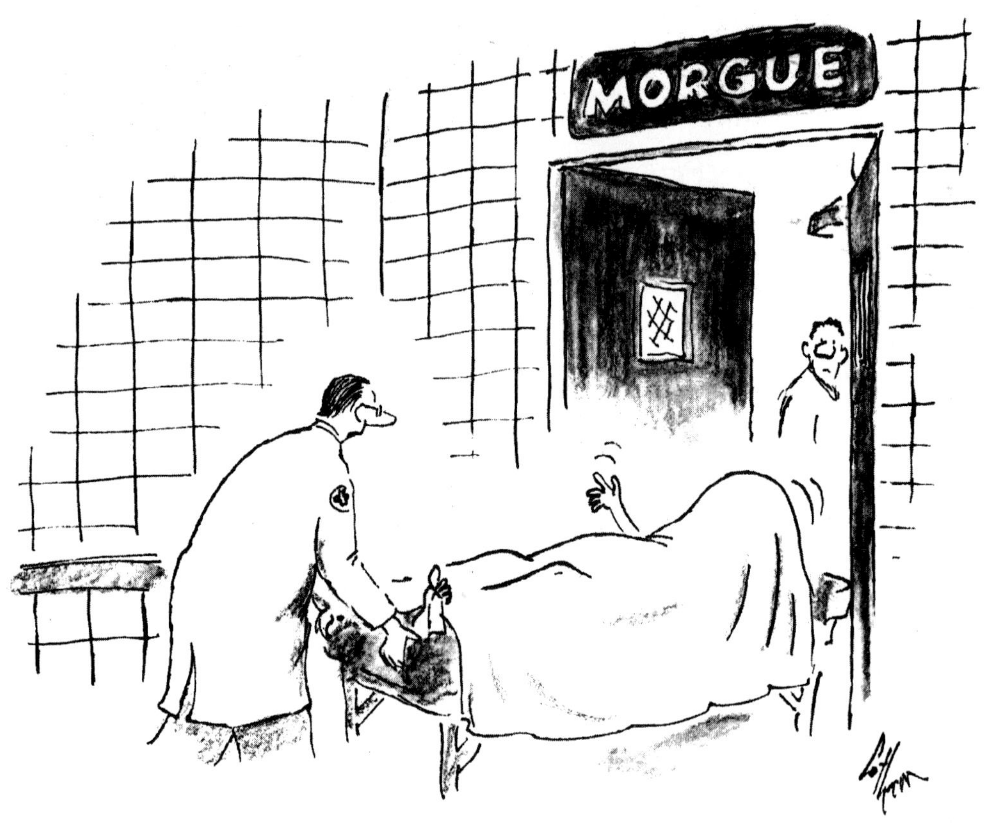

"Okay! I'll pay!"

7.

Anatomy of an Illness

Diagnostic odds and ends

Symptoms from Outer Space

Medical sideshows

Dr. Strangelove presents

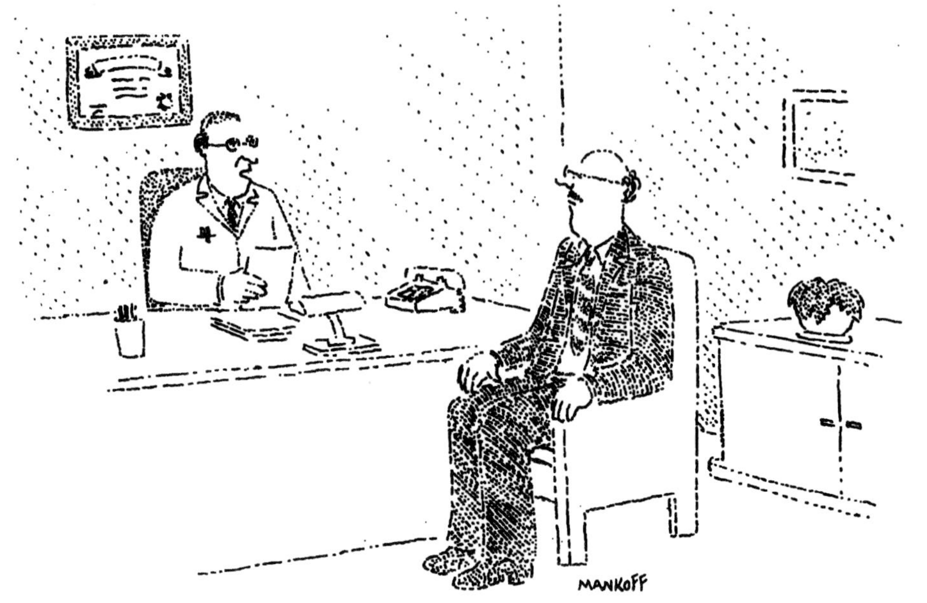

"Well, Phil, after years of vague complaints and imaginary ailments, we finally have something to work with."

HERMAN®

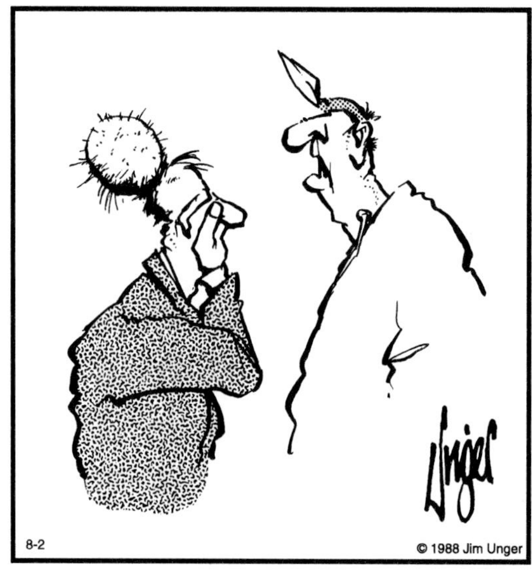

"You should never stifle a sneeze!"

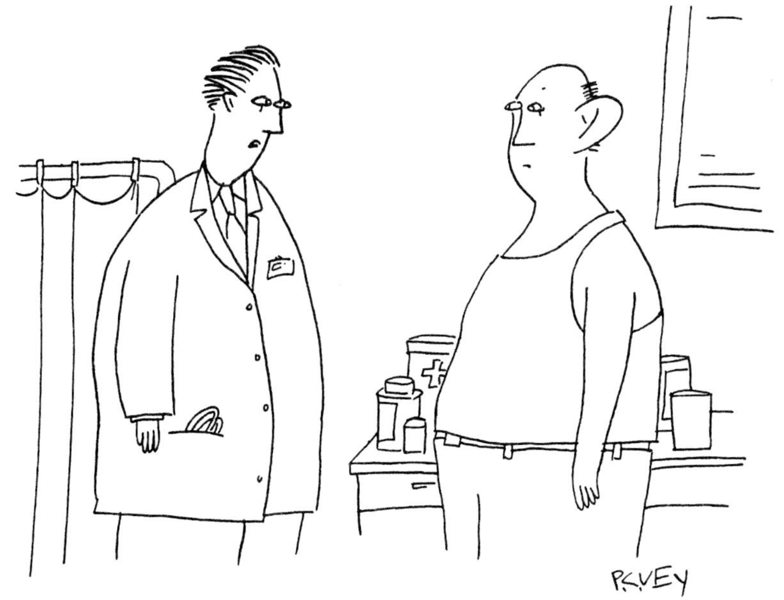

"No, big ears are not a sign of virility."

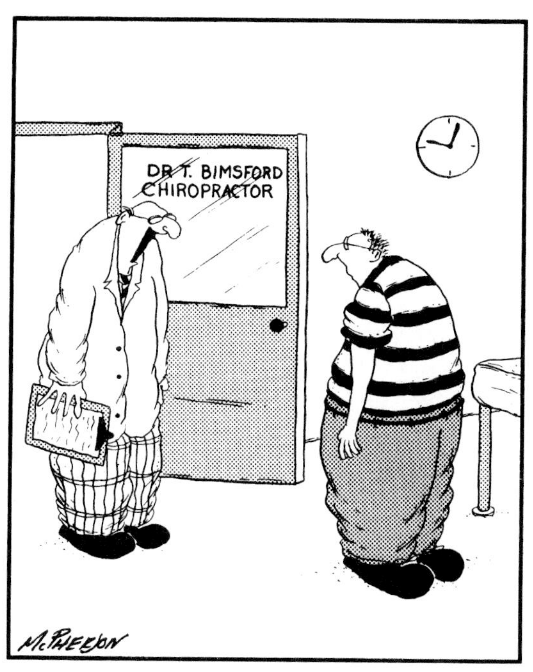

"Well now, Mr. Fenderson, what seems to be the problem?"

HERMAN®

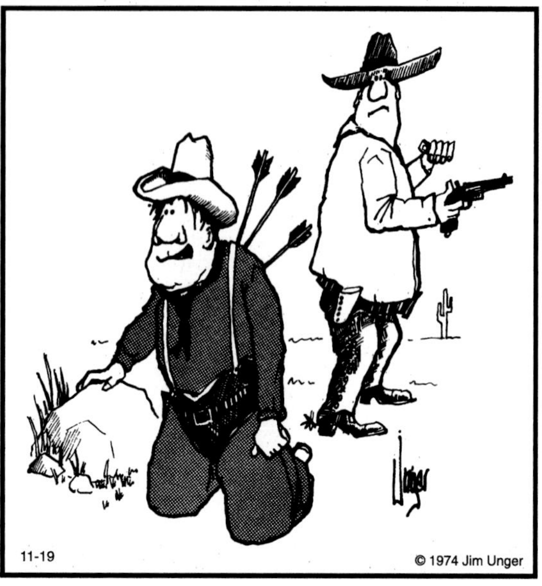

"They've cured my arthritis!"

HERMAN®

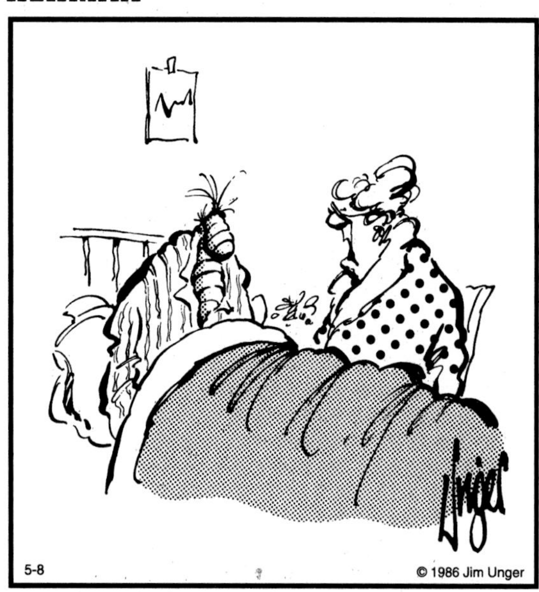

"How was I supposed to know you were in the shower when I flushed?"

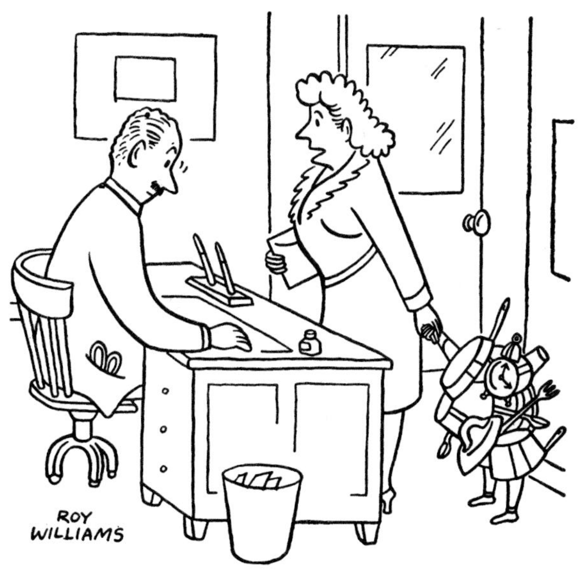

"It's Maureen, doctor. She just swallowed a magnet."

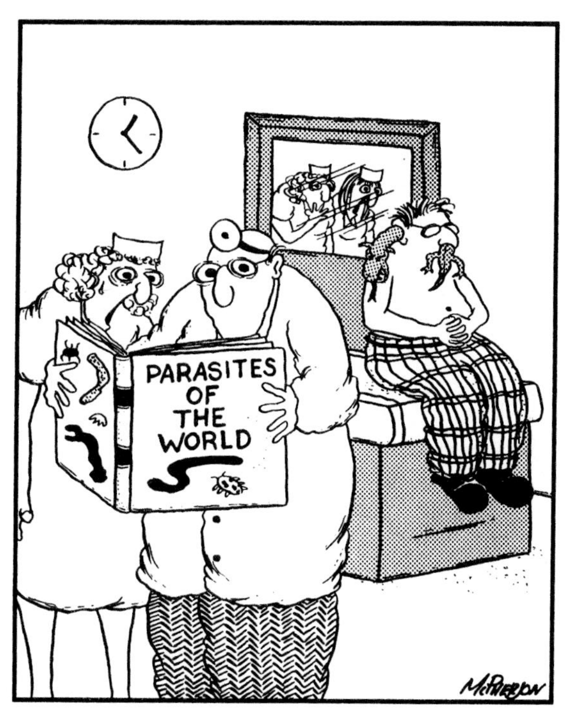

McPHERSON

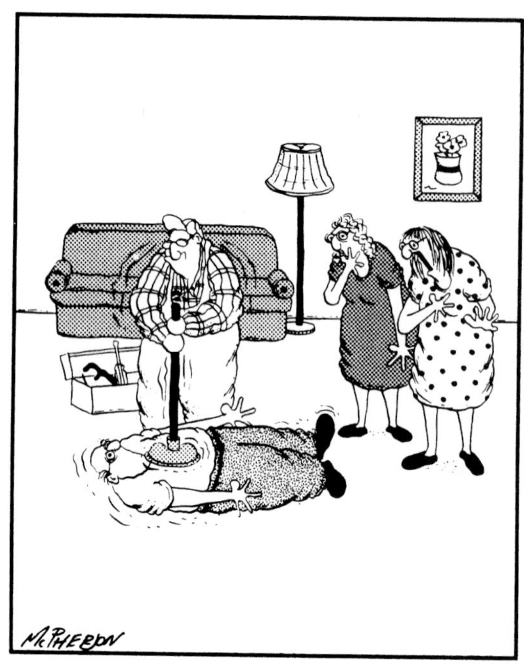

"Thank heavens the plumber knows CPR!"

McPHERSON

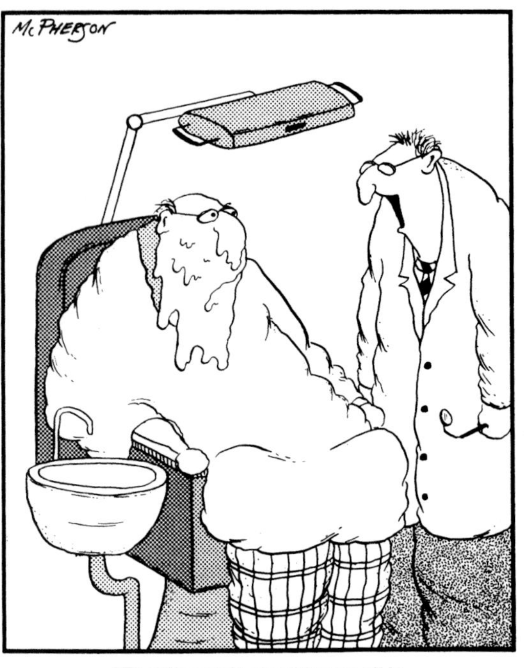

"That Novocain should wear off in two or three days."

CHARLIE
THE PLACEBOS DON'T SEEM TO BE WORKING, DOCTOR...
I WAS AFRAID OF THAT-TOMORROW MORNING AT 9:30 I'LL PRETEND I'M GOING TO OPERATE.
11-6

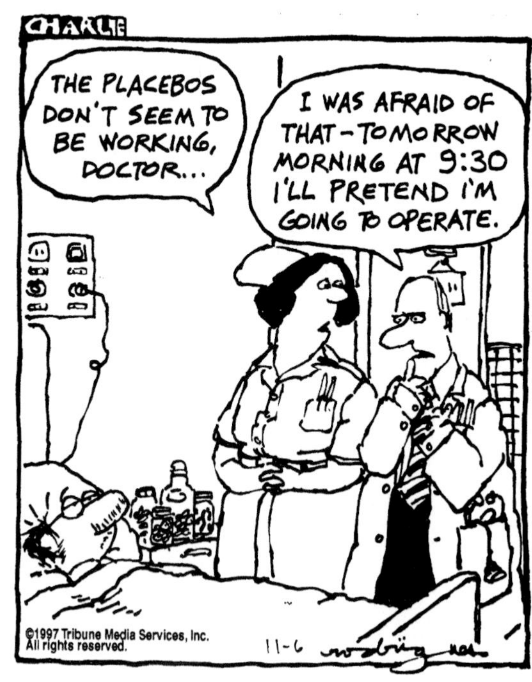

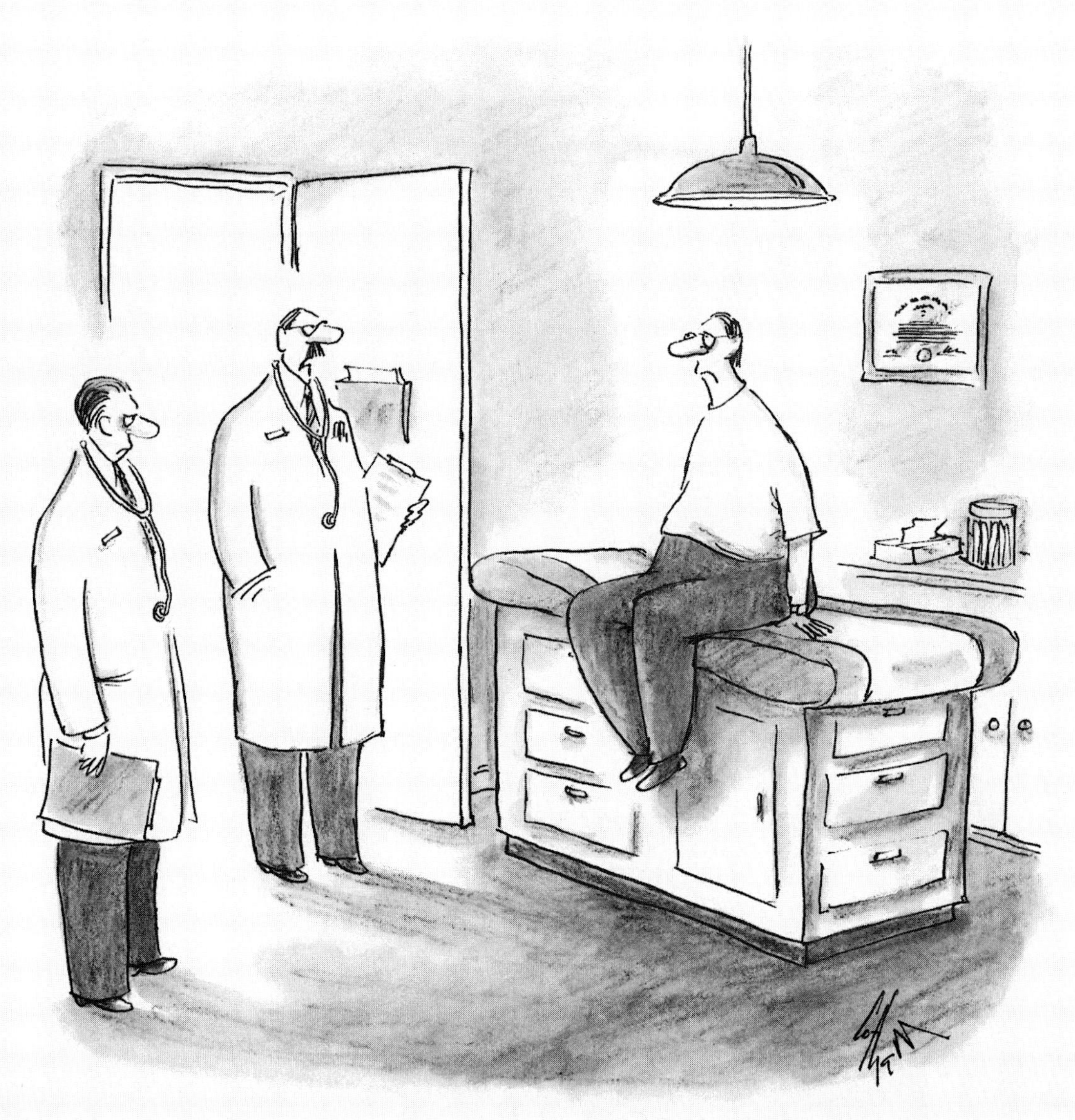

"May I cross-examine the patient?"

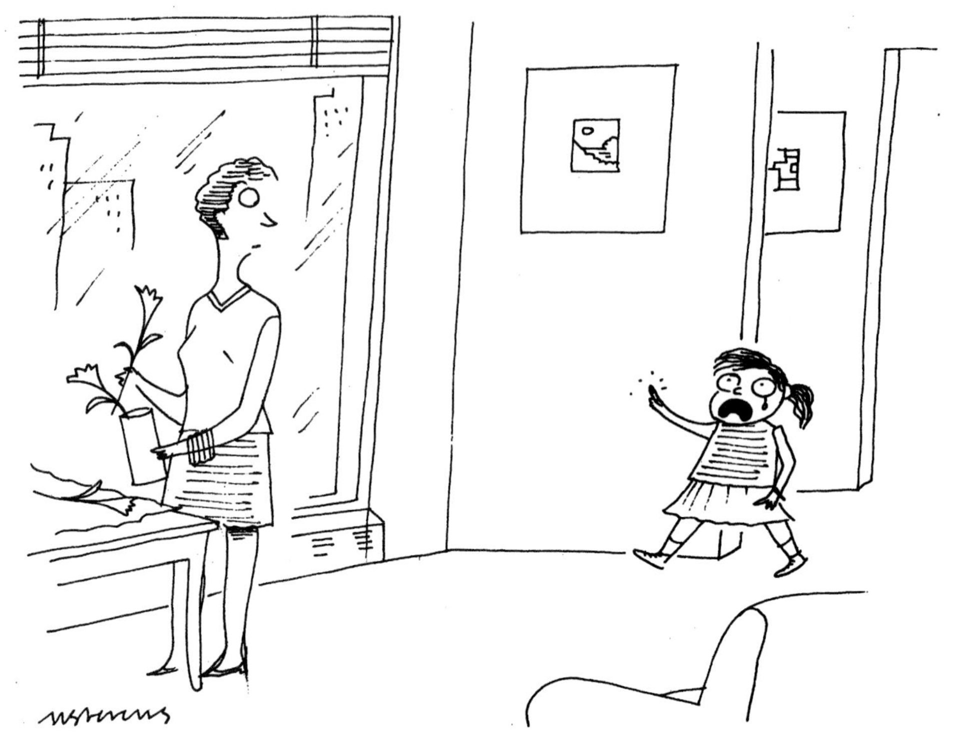

"Health-care!"

HERMAN®

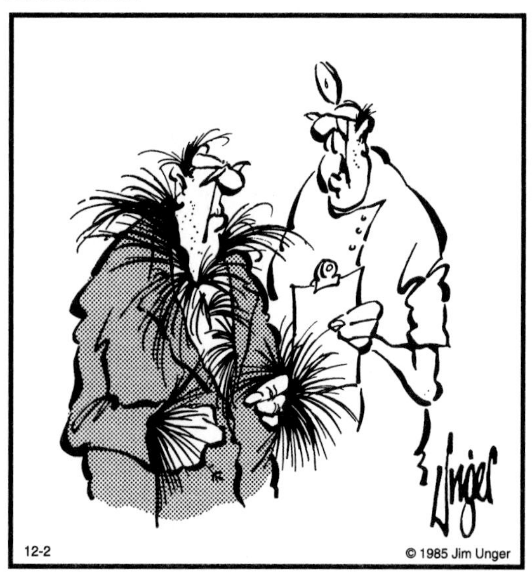

"Classic hay fever."

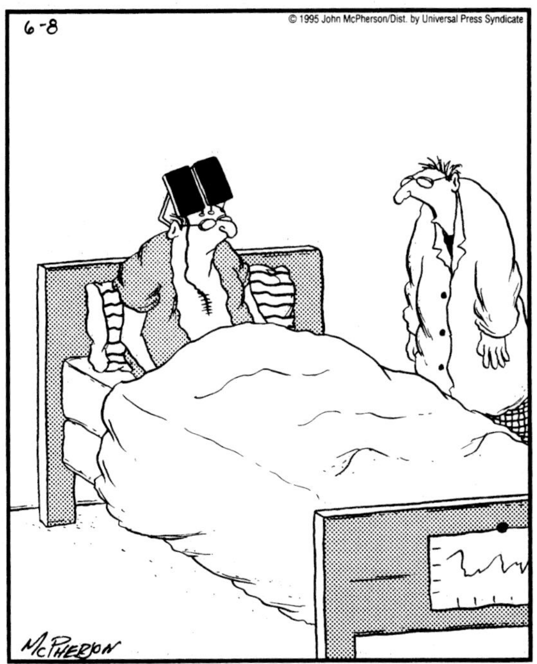

"If you start to feel dizzy or weak, get outside immediately. Your new pacemaker is solar-powered."

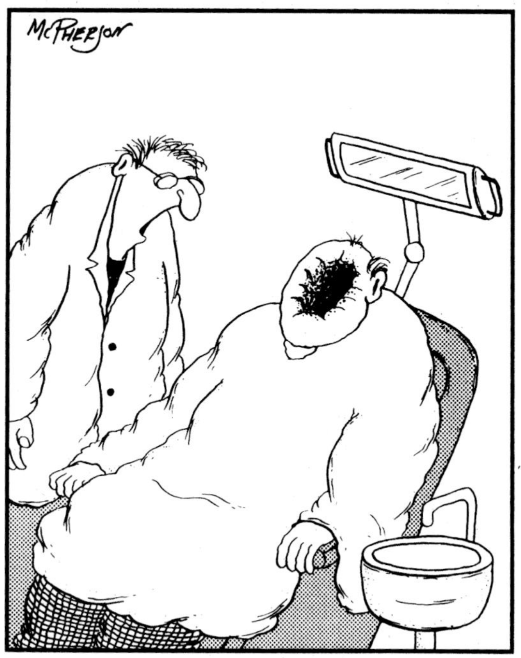

"You let that cavity go far too long."

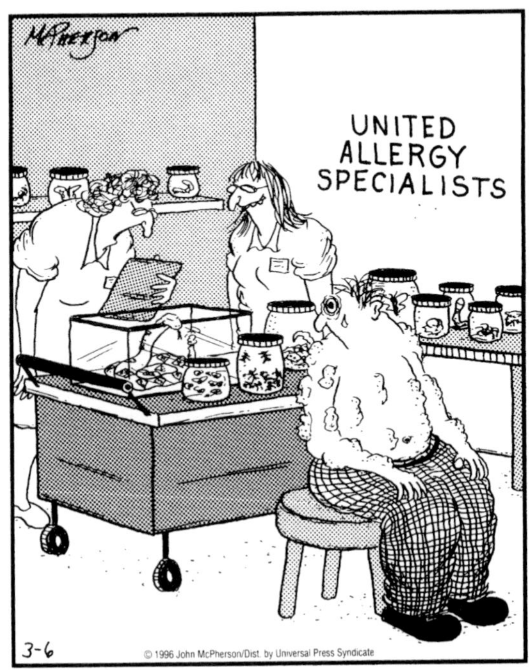

"Well, let's see. He's positive for hay fever, negative for mildew, positive for poison ivy, positive for bee stings, positive for poison sumac. Let's see how he does with the fire ants."

REAL LIFE ADVENTURES by Gary Wise and Lance Aldrich

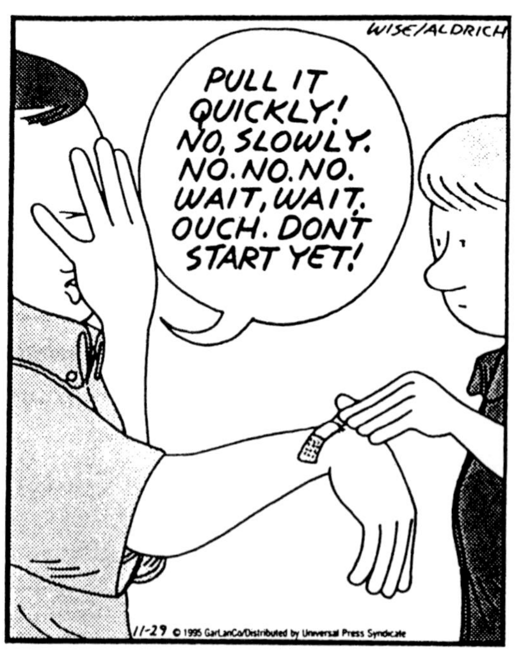

The most feared and dreaded medical procedure there is.

8.

Nursing Your Wounds

Me and sympathy

Bedside encounters

The good, the bad, the ridiculous

Don't worry

HERMAN®

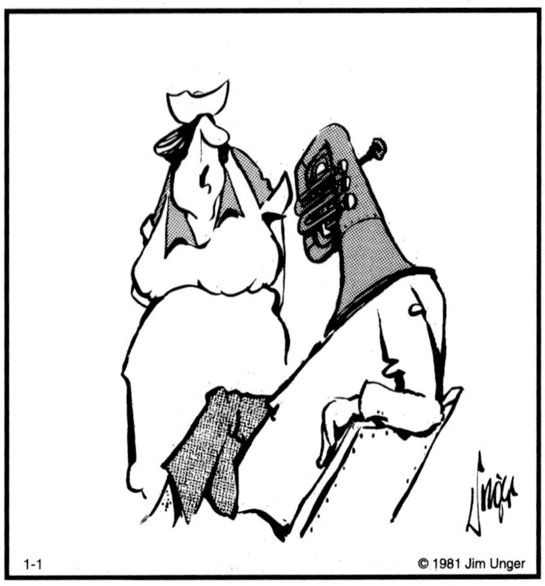

"The doctor won't be long. Are you sure you wouldn't like a cup of coffee?"

HERMAN®

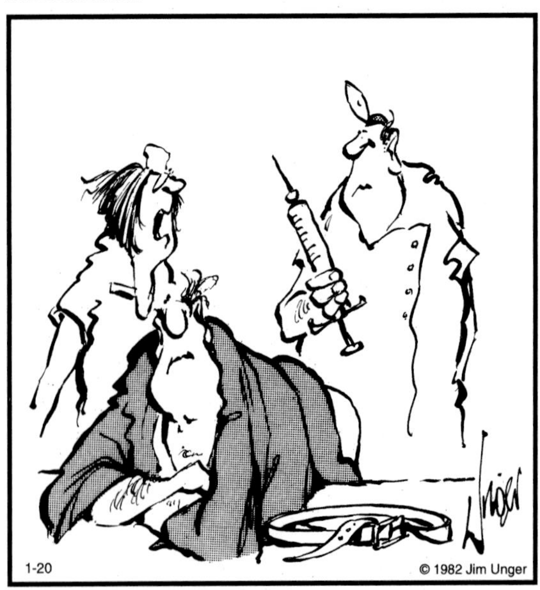

"Oh please! I promise I won't mess it up like last time."

TRY TO HOLD THE NEEDLE STEADY, DANNY. THAT'S GOOD ENOUGH.
ZZZAP!
McPHERSON

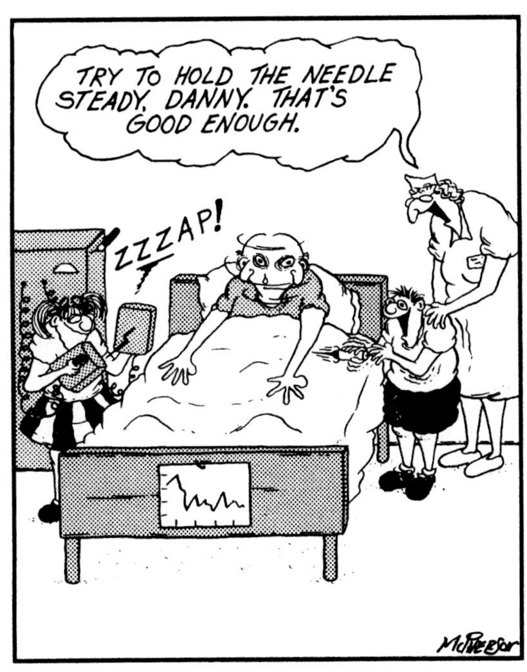

Take Your Child to Work Day at Fernview Hospital.

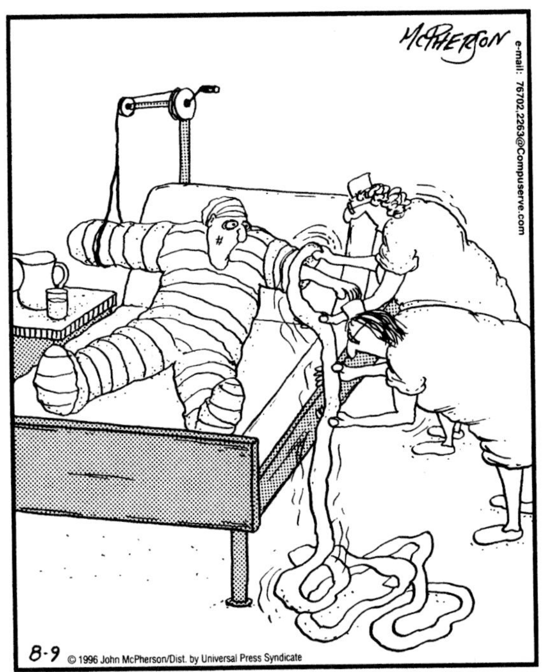

"Sorry to have to redo this, but Carol Ann is pretty sure that her missing earring is in here somewhere."

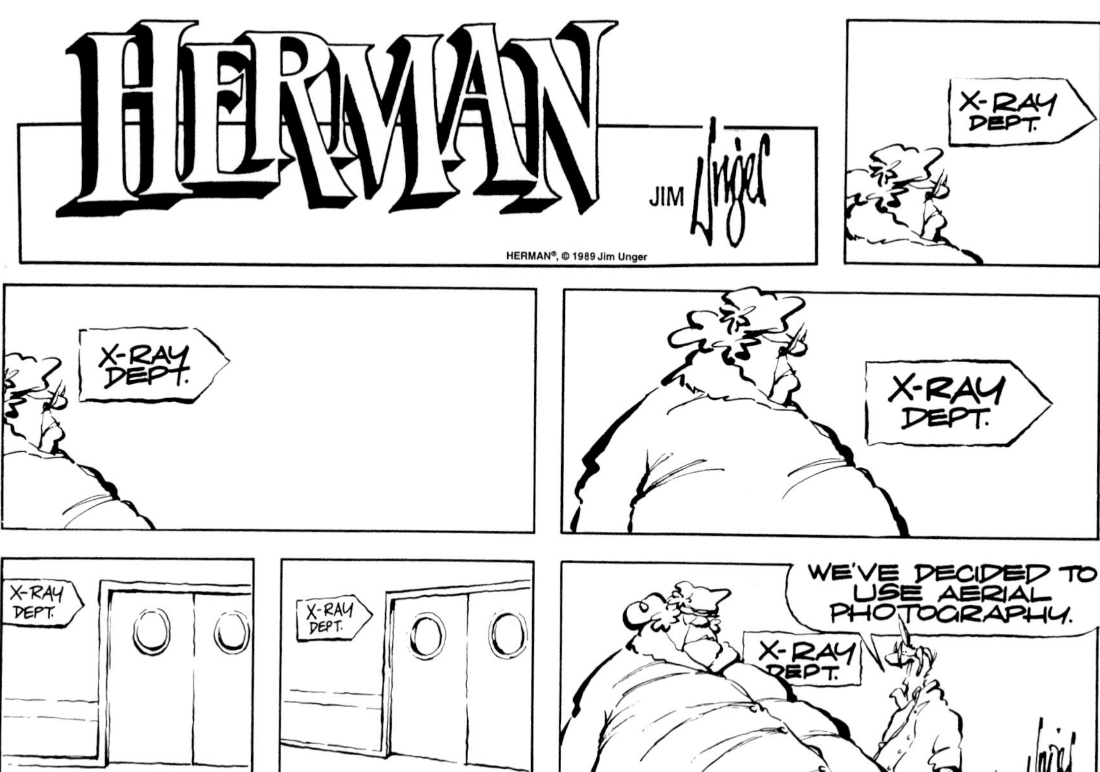
HERMAN
JIM Unger
HERMAN®, © 1989 Jim Unger
X-RAY DEPT.
X-RAY DEPT.
X-RAY DEPT.
X-RAY DEPT.
X-RAY DEPT.
WE'VE DECIDED TO USE AERIAL PHOTOGRAPHY.
X-RAY DEPT.
3/12 Unger

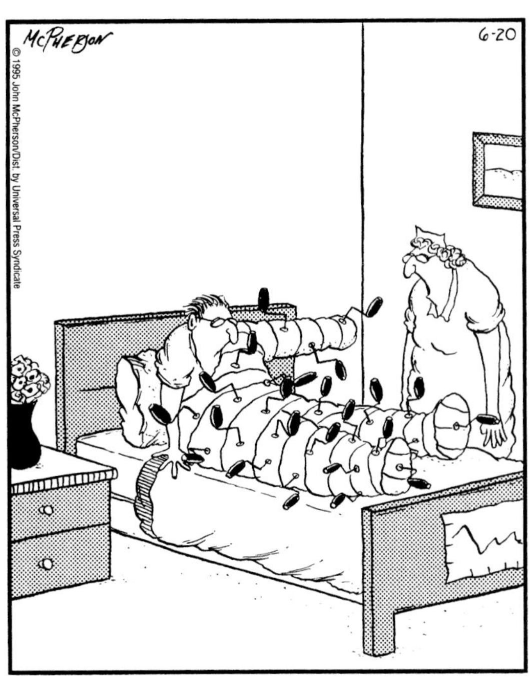

"If you get an itch, just turn whichever one of these cranks is closest to it."

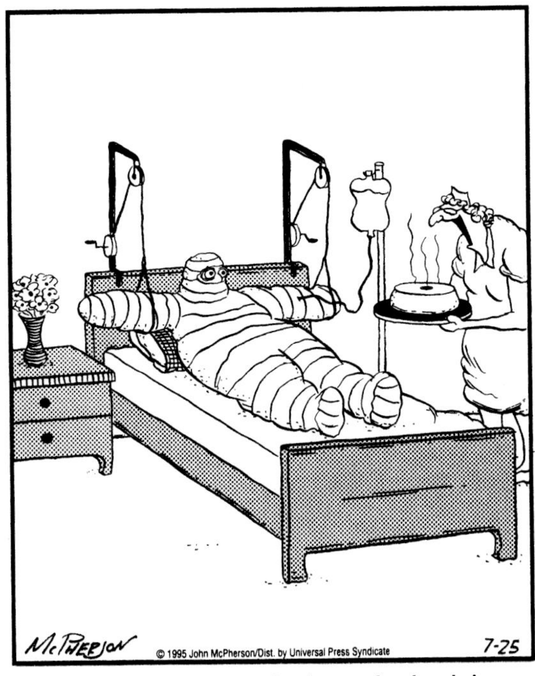

"Here you go! T-bone steak, mashed potatoes and fresh asparagus! Whoops! What am I doing? This is for Mr. Cagner in room 173."

HERMAN®

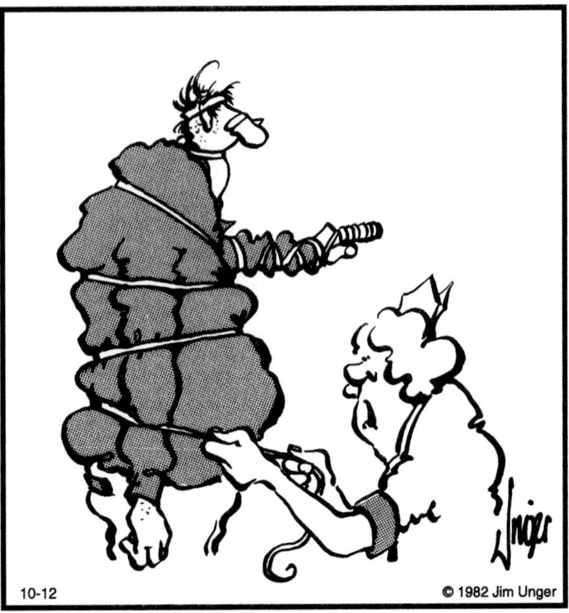

"I wonder why they make these finger bandages so long?"

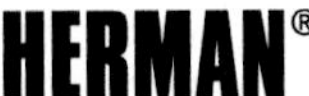

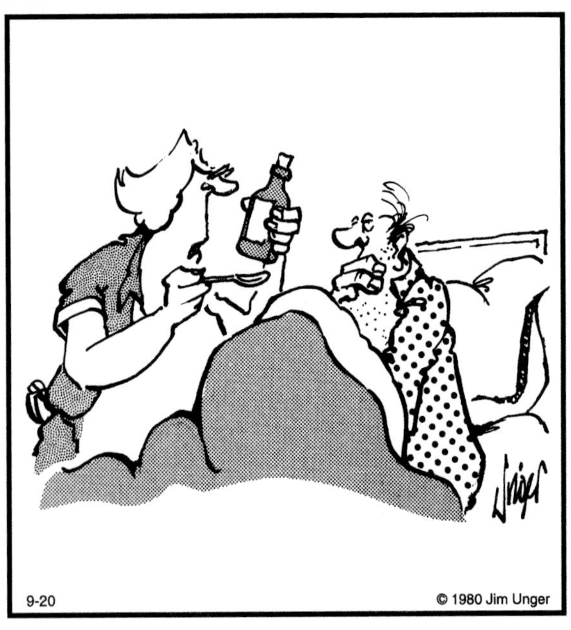

"My mistake. I'm supposed to rub it on your chest."

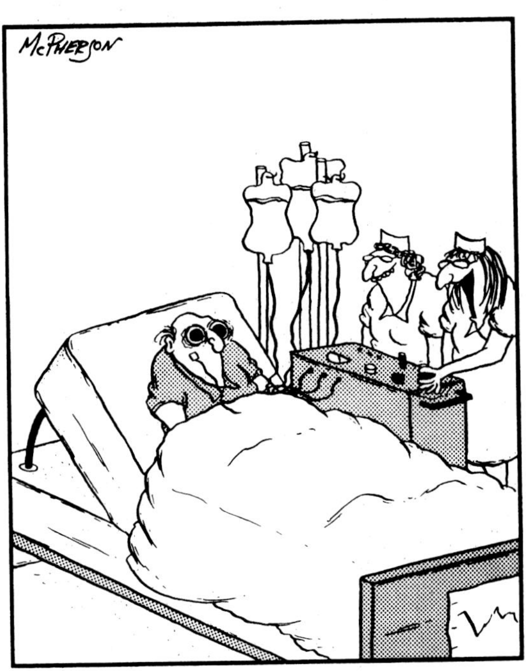

"Hey, Carol! Look how big his eyes get when you turn this blue dial *way* up!"

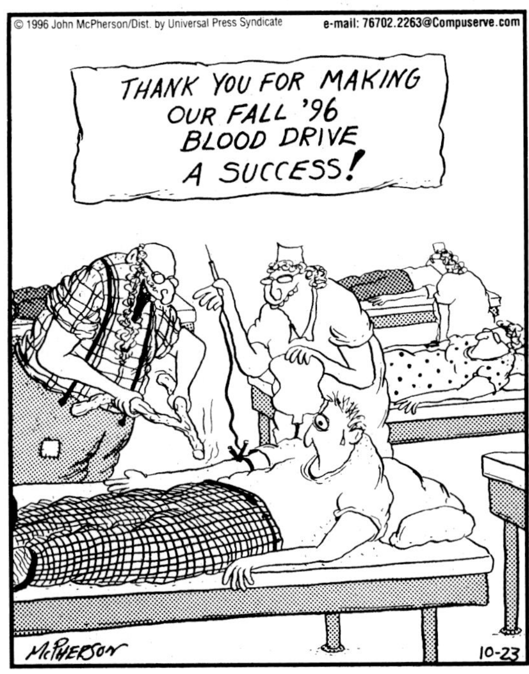

"I'd say you want to stick it right about there! Yep, there's a real gusher right where that mole is!"

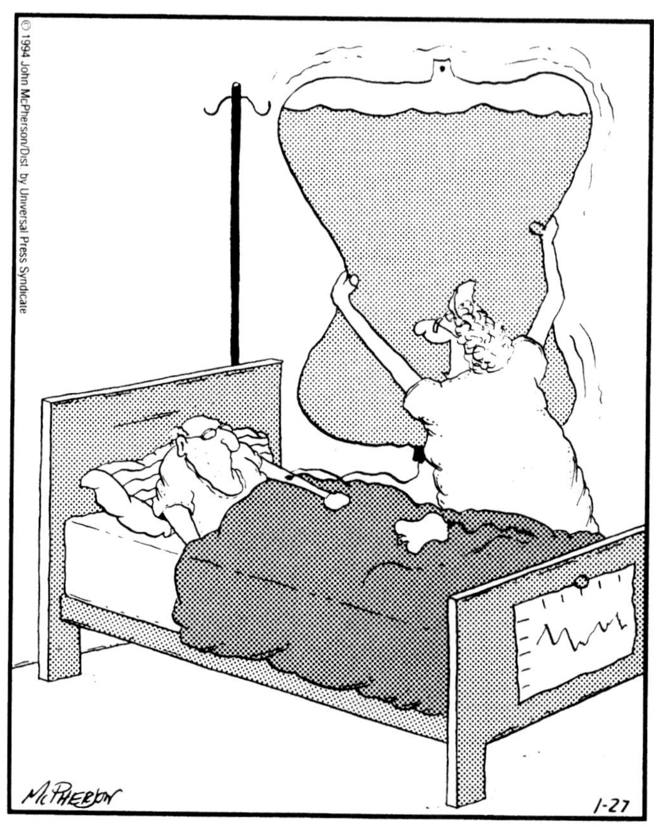

"I'll be going to the Bahamas for a week starting tomorrow. This should tide you over 'til I get back."

9. A Bitter Pill to Swallow

Funny pills, Sad pills

Side effects on the wild side

Medication madness

Reactions and Interactions

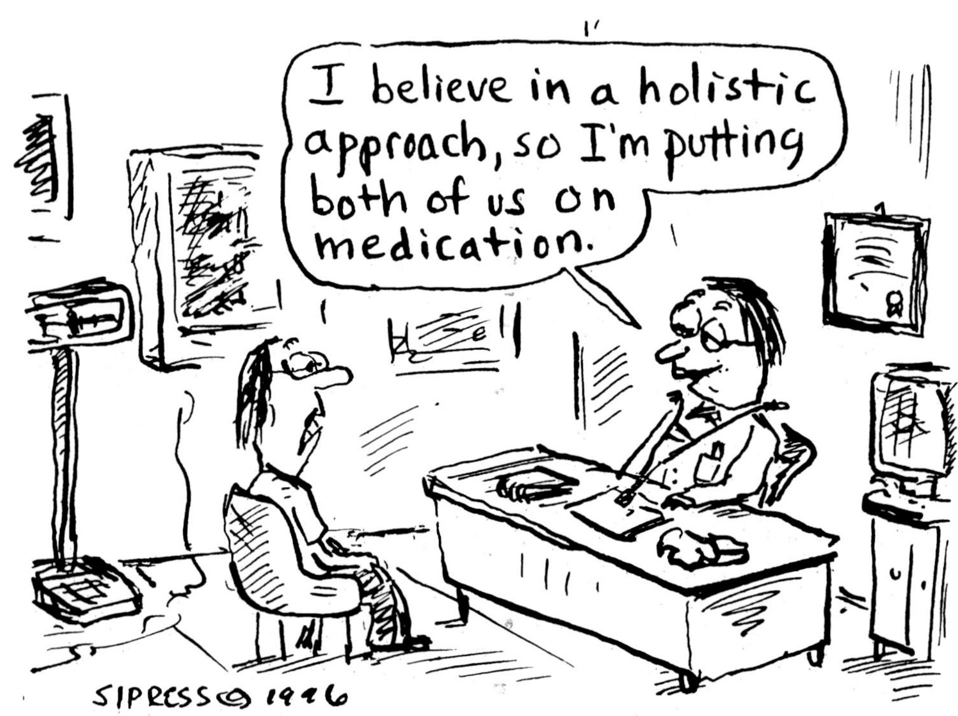
I believe in a holistic approach, so I'm putting both of us on medication.
SIPRESS © 1996

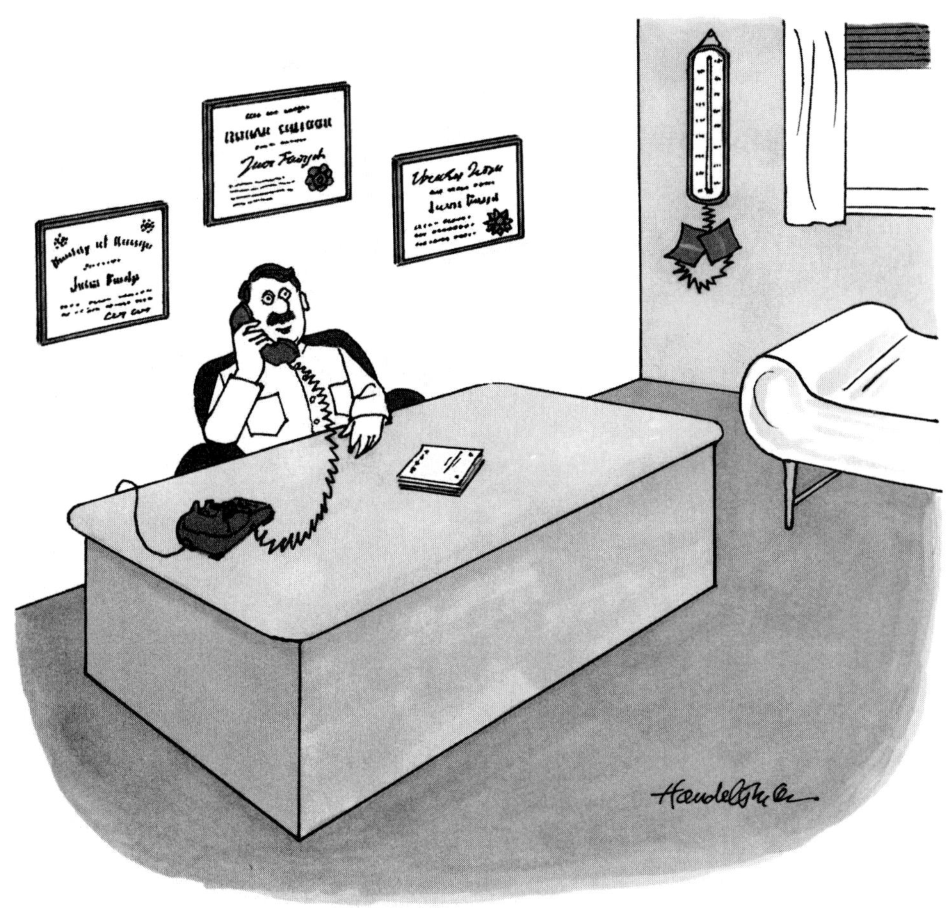

"Before we try assisted suicide, Mrs. Rose, let's give the aspirin a chance."

HERMAN®

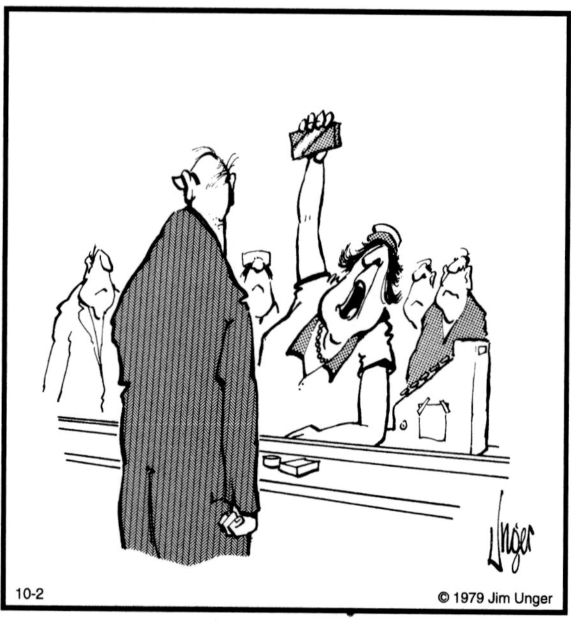

"HARRY... HOW MUCH ARE THESE LAXATIVE PILLS?"

HERMAN®

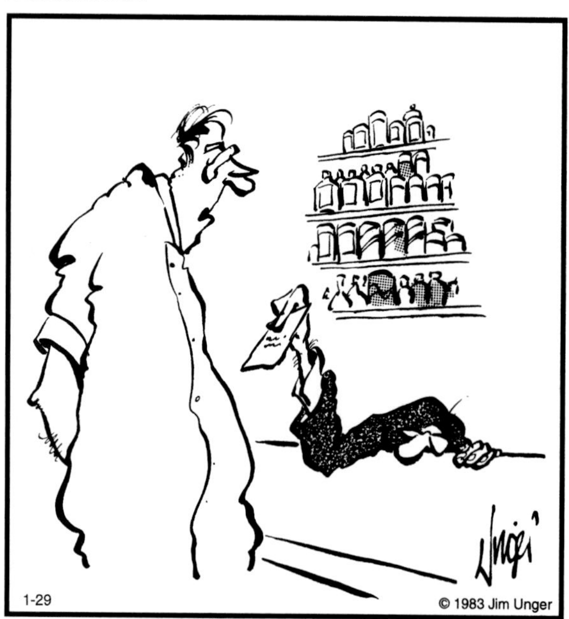

"I'm sorry, we're out of 'Multivitamins Plus Iron.'"

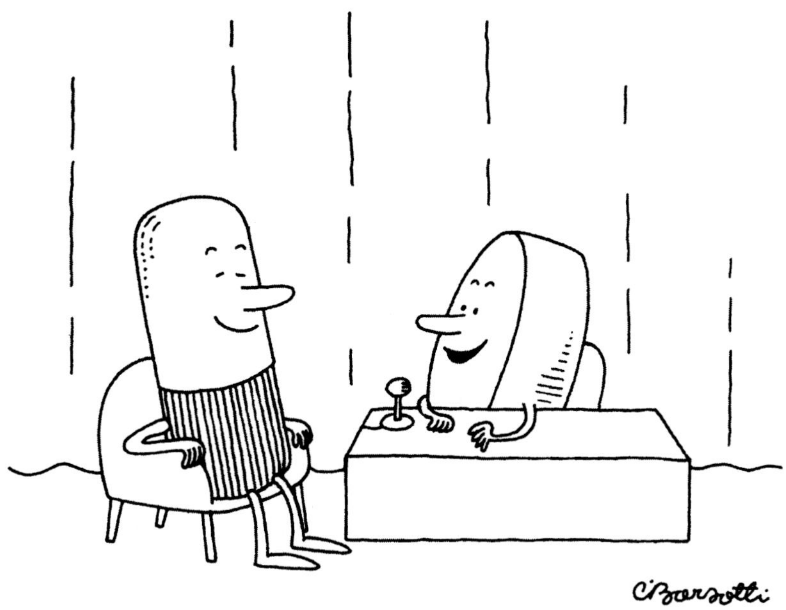

"I understand they've uncovered some weird new side effects since you were here last."

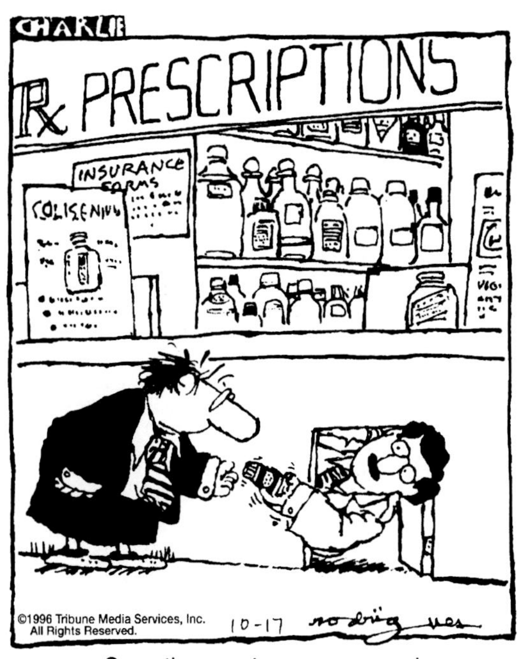

Sometime next year we expect
it to be sold **over** the counter."

—THIS IS A RELEASE FORM WE'D LIKE YOU TO SIGN. SHOULD YOU BECOME DELIRIOUS FROM THE MEDICATION & BEGIN BABBLING, THIS GIVES US THE RIGHT TO RECORD YOU AND USE IT ON OUR NEXT COMEDY CD, *THE BEST FROM MERCY HOSPITAL, VOLUME II.*
HOSPITAL ADMISSIONS
HTTP://WWW.VDGI.COM/BIZARRO
BIZARRO © DAN PIRARO · 1996

N-E-O-C-I-N-E. NEOCINE. WELL, I'VE NEVER HEARD OF IT, BUT I'LL PRESCRIBE A TWO-WEEK DOSAGE OF IT AND SEE IF IT DOES HIM ANY GOOD.
OUIJA BOARD
McPHERSON
© 1996 John McPherson/Dist. by Universal Press Syndicate
1-9

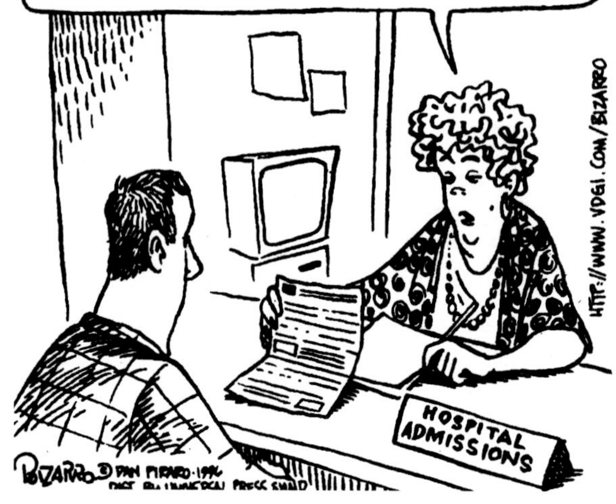

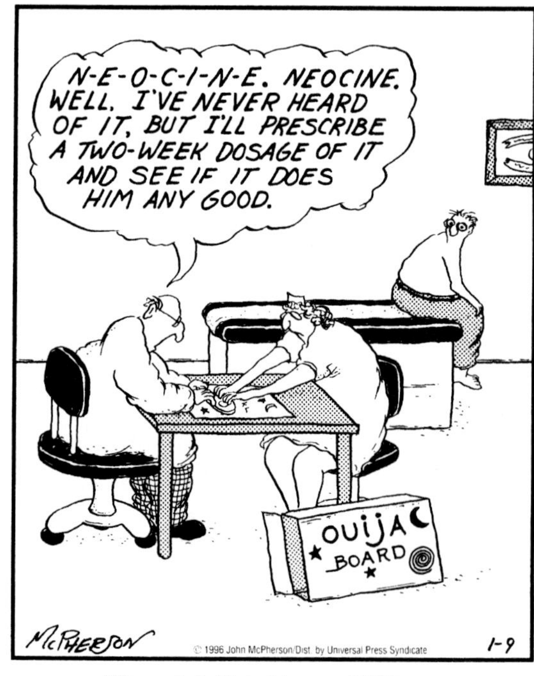

Wayne's faith in his new HMO was eroding quickly.

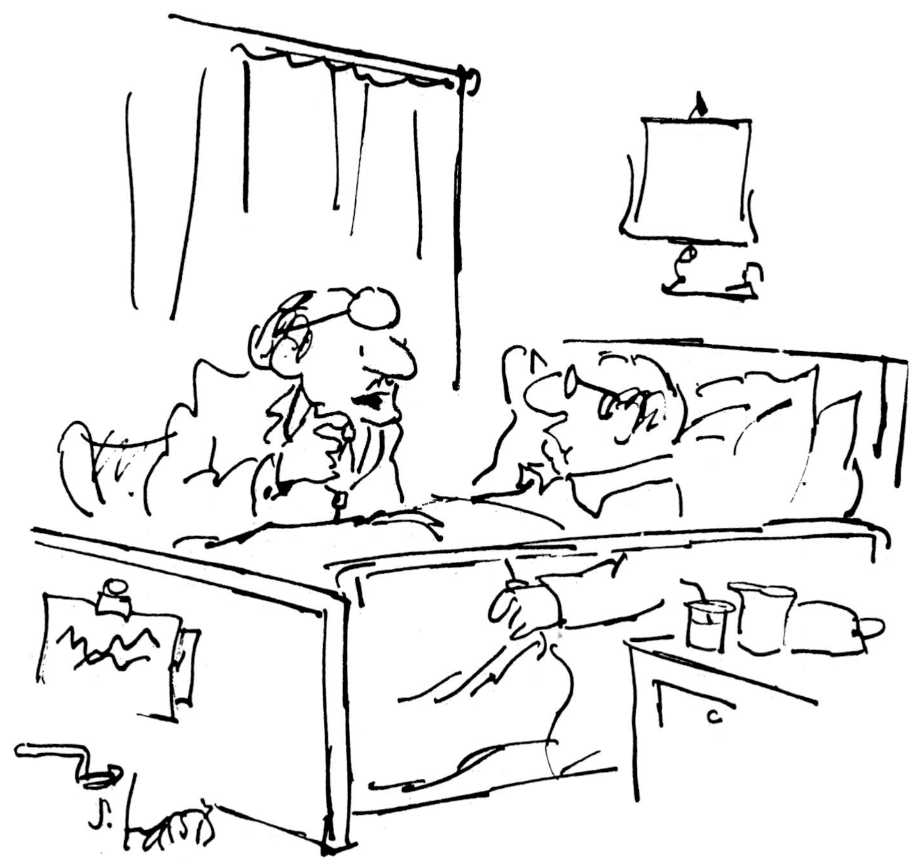

"Fewer than one in ten thousand — something like one in fourteen thousand — gets these side effects. Hardly anybody gets these side effects. They're extremely rare. You should be very proud."

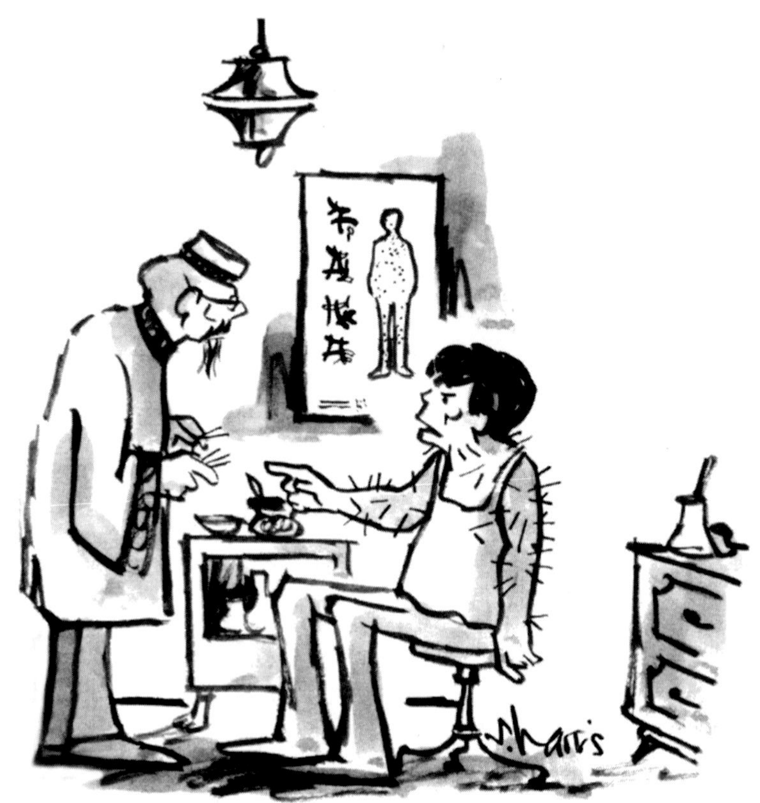

"Enough acupuncture — get me a couple of aspirin."

HI, ED. I NEED A DECONGESTANT, SOMETHING FOR CHICKEN POX, AND SOMETHING FOR AN EAR INFECTION.
PHARMACY

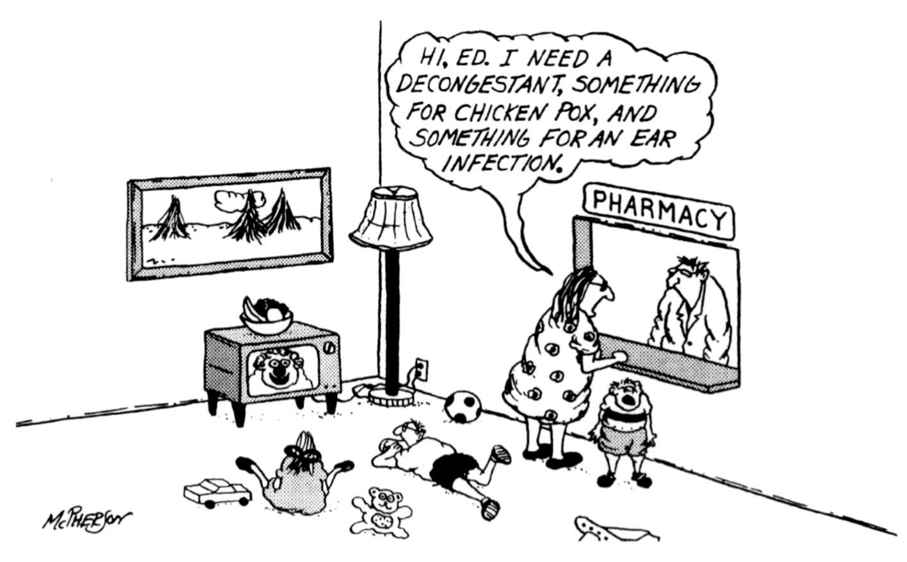

For the sake of convenience, parents with several children are opting to have in-home pharmacists.

PRESCRIPTION DRUGS '96

PRESERVE®
For people who are O.K. with feeling more or less the way they do today.
FREEZE®
A pill for people who would just like things to not get any worse.
MESA®
A pharmaceutical scenic overlook for those on the downward slope.

LIBBY REID/GIDEON BOSKER

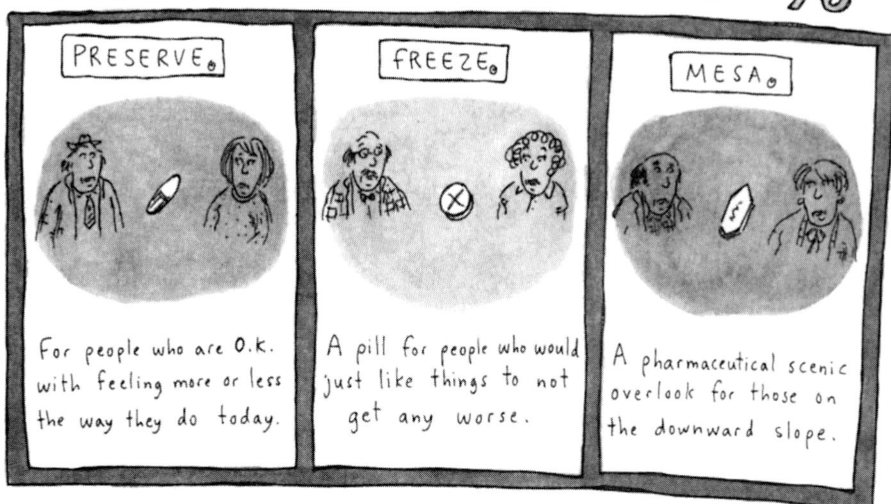

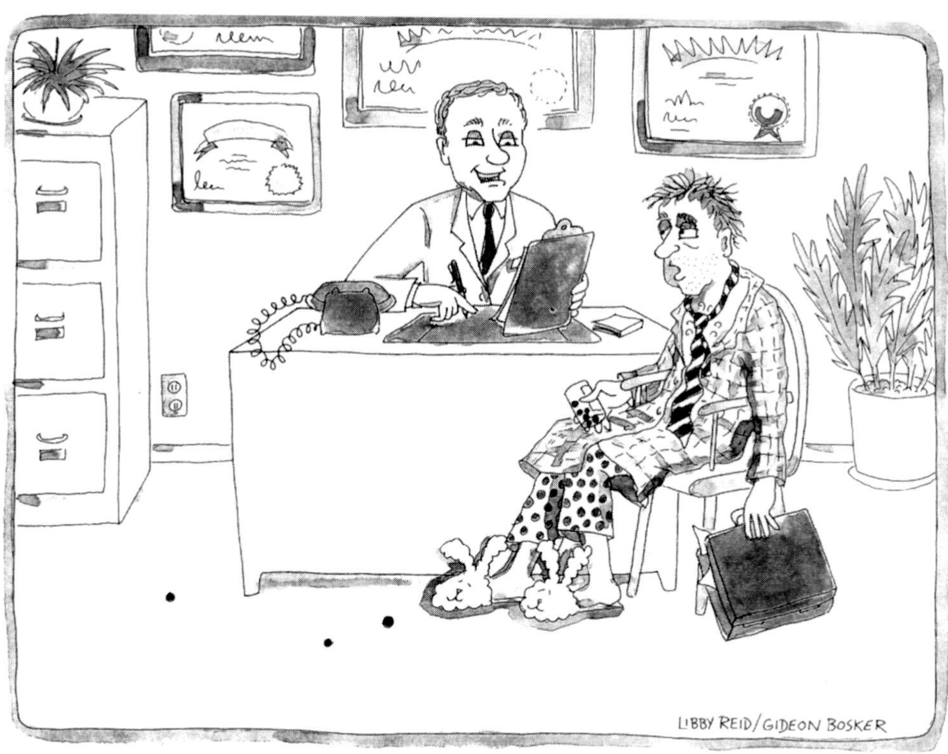

Not to worry, Mr. Salem, all medications can produce mild side effects. The question is, have they affected your quality-of-life?

①
The first medication I'm prescribing is for the headaches.
②
Then I'm prescribing something for the swelling and something else for the over-all problem...
③
And finally, I'll be prescribing some valium.
Valium? What's the valium for?
It's to help you cope with the cost of the other medications.
SIPRESS

PHARMACY
McPHERSON

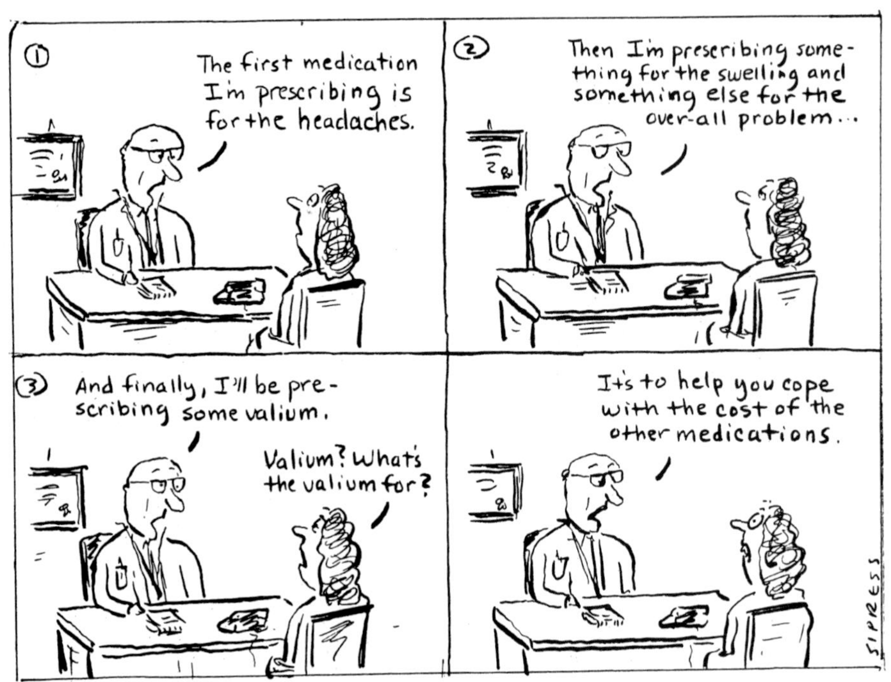

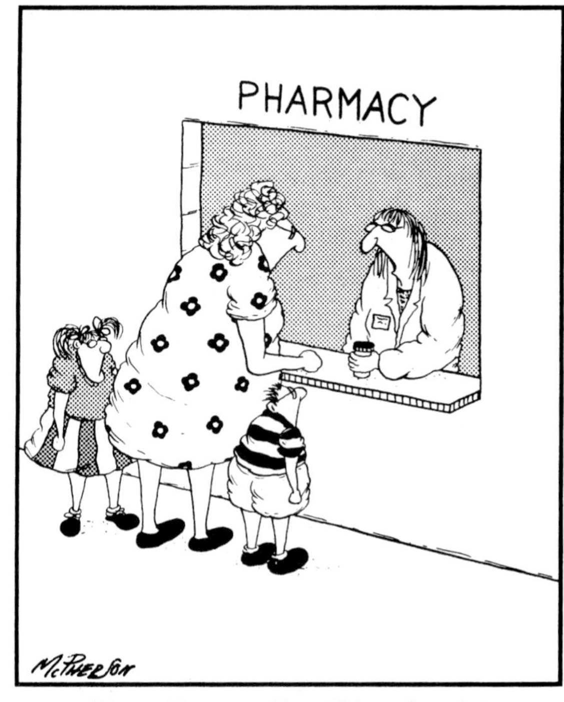

"These pills come with a child-proof cap, but as an added precaution they're manufactured to look exactly like lima beans."

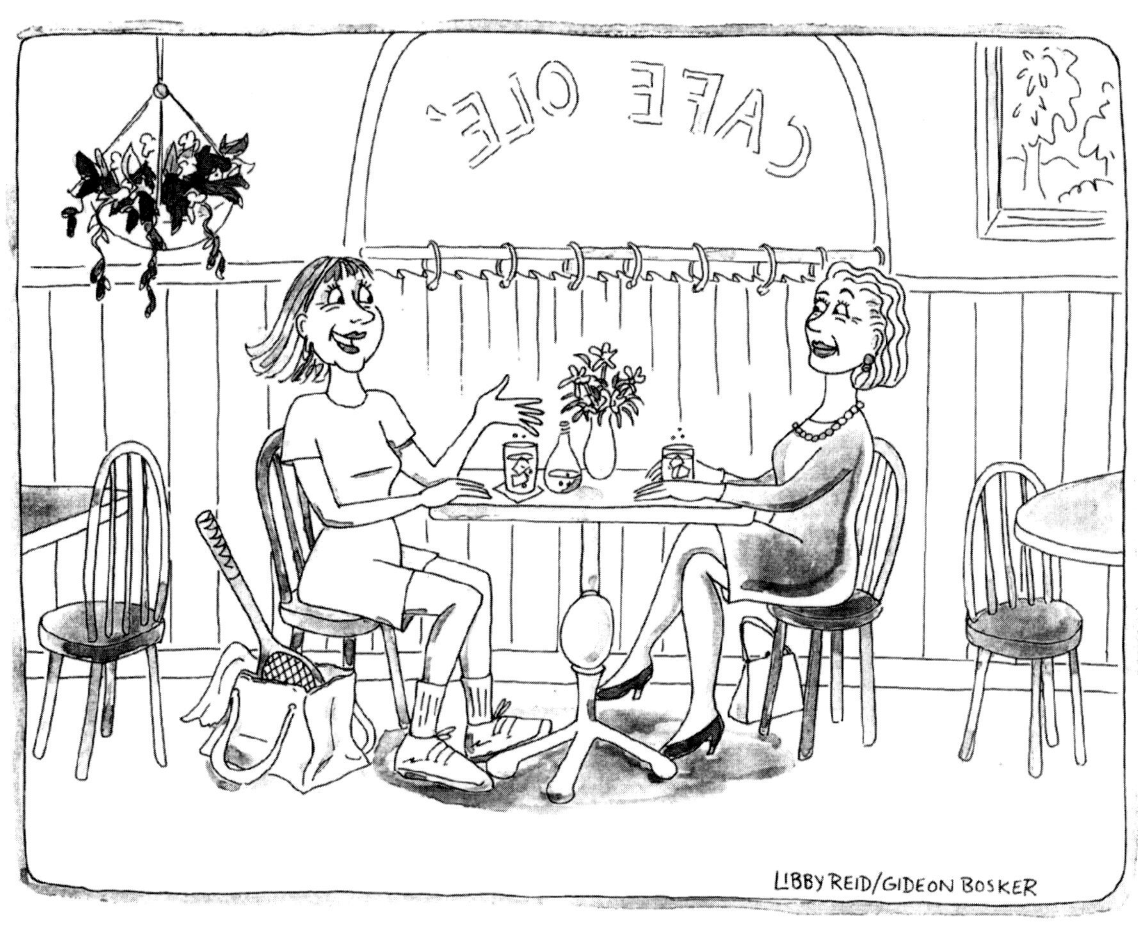

That's right, Eleanor, I divorced Harry and replaced him with estrogen.

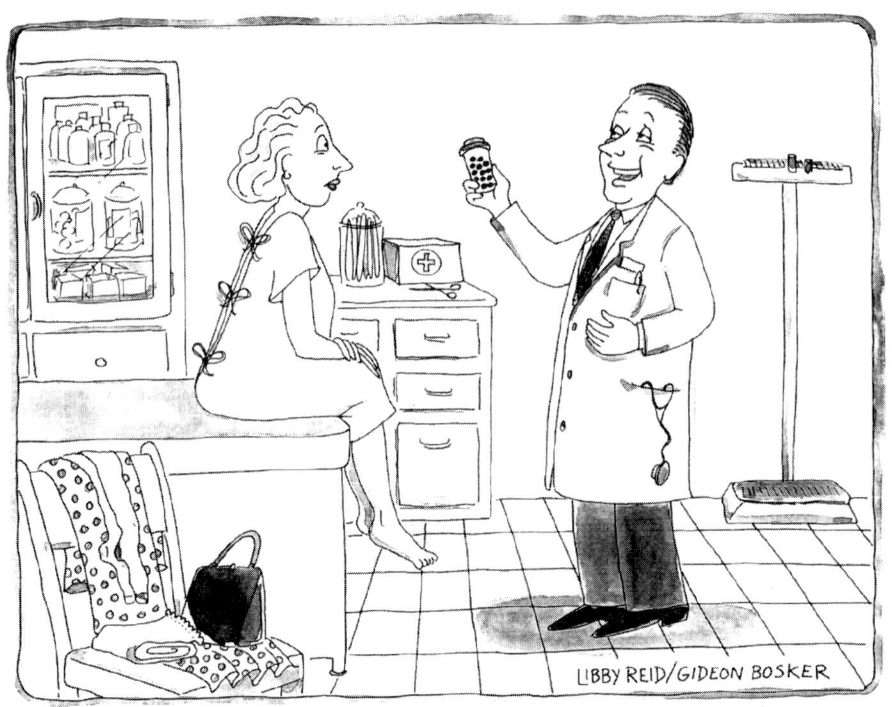

Be sure you take these pills with food. And may I suggest seared Ahi tuna, baby new potatoes, and Tiramisu for dessert?

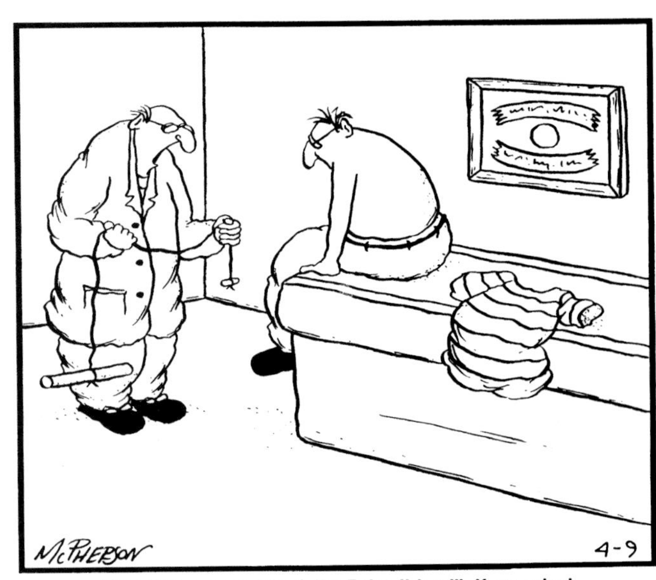

"OK, listen *very* carefully. Take this pill. If you start to feel numbness in your legs or have trouble pronouncing vowels, pull it out immediately."

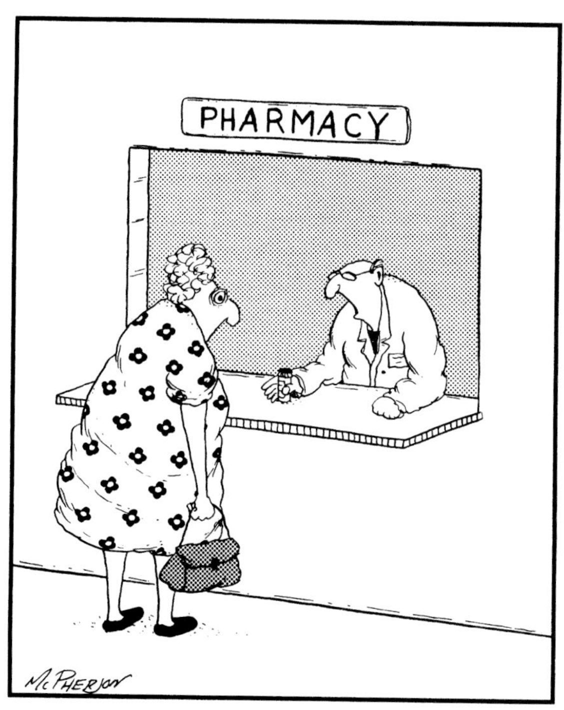

"I had trouble reading your doctor's handwriting, but I think I figured it out. However, if you start to drool uncontrollably or gain more than 15 pounds in a week, stop taking them."

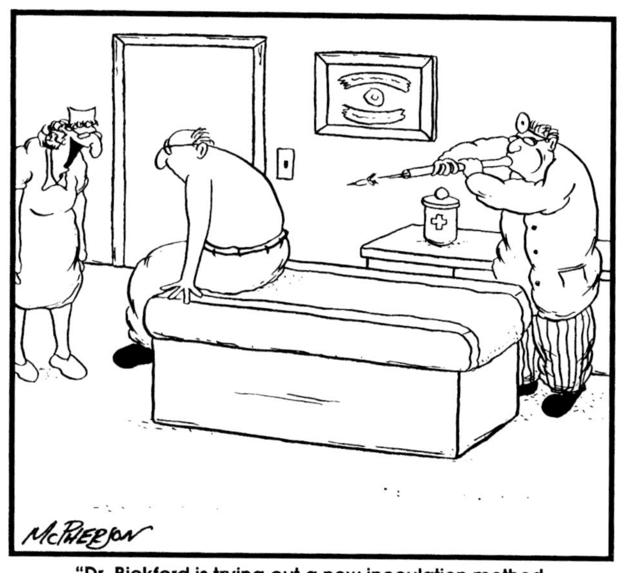

"Dr. Bickford is trying out a new inoculation method he found out about when he was traveling in Borneo."

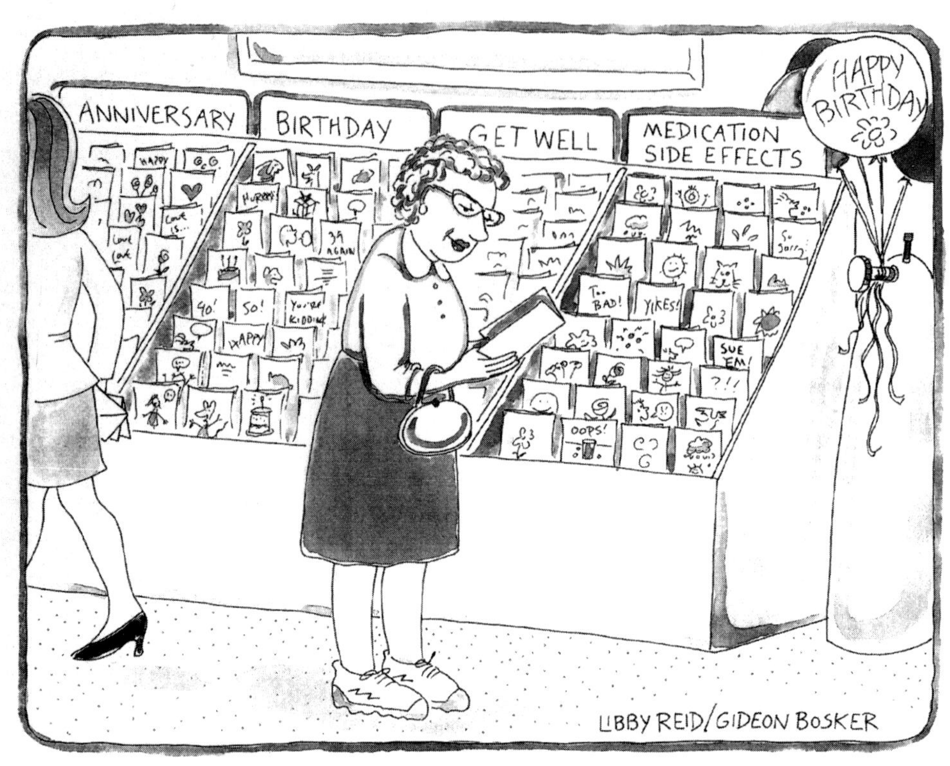

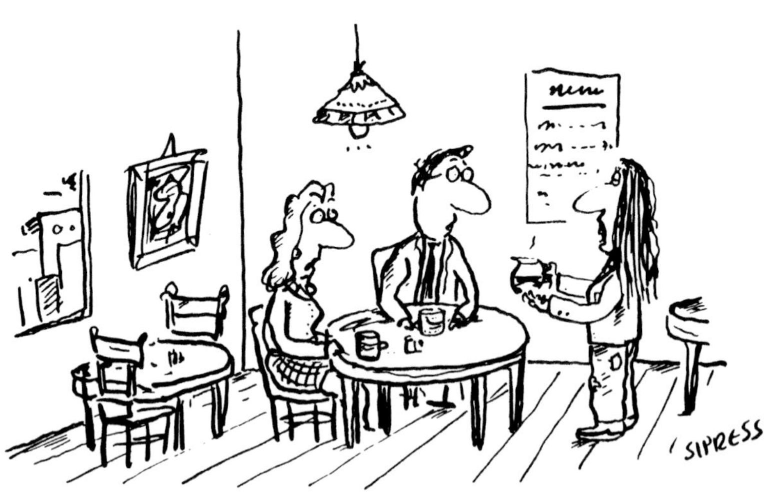

I'm afraid we're out of decaf tonight, but I can offer you regular coffee and a couple of valium.

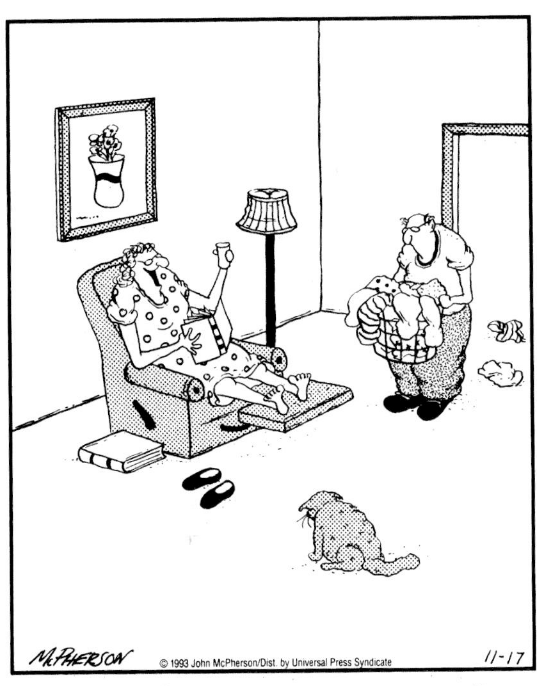

"I *told* you! I can't do the laundry *or* use the stove! The allergy medicine I'm on says not to operate heavy equipment."

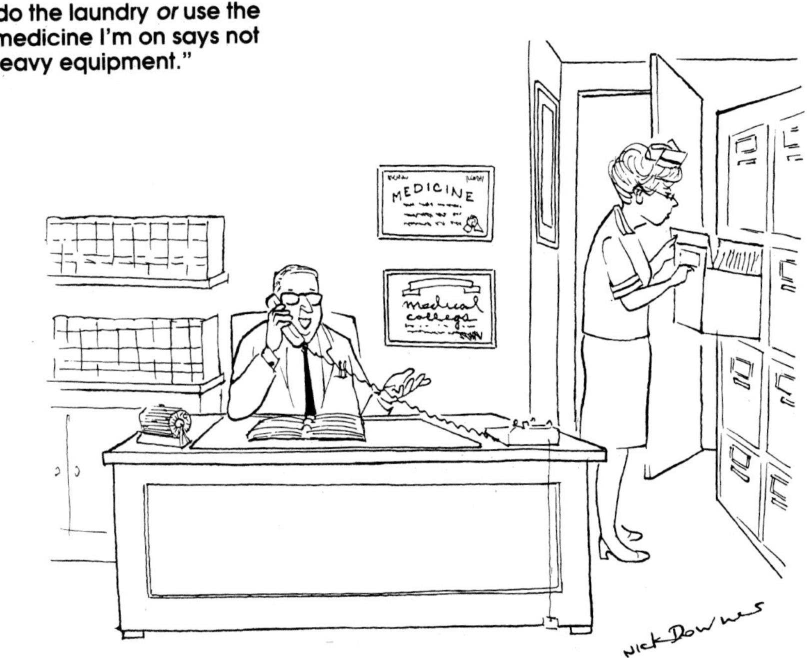

"Of course you're furious over the price of your medication, Mr. Grimwald — that's one of its side effects."

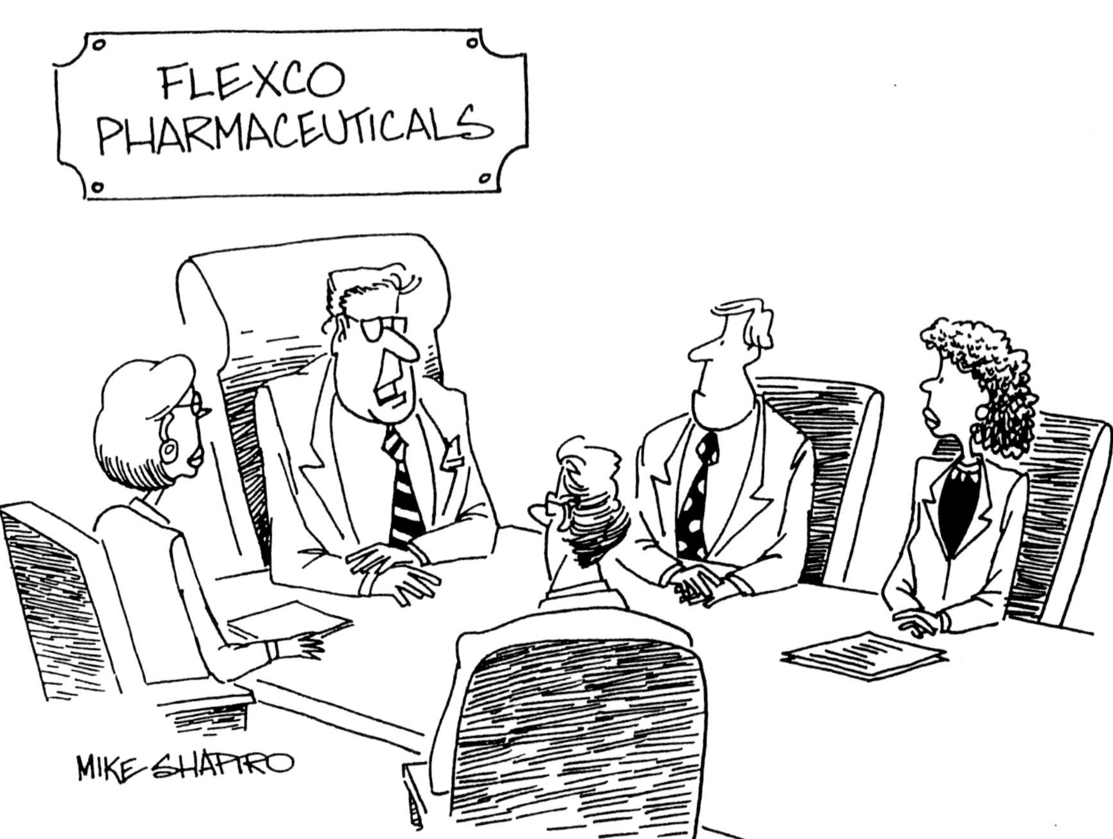

"Bad news, people. The latest research indicates that laughter really is the best medicine."

10.

From Here to Maternity

Nursery room humor

Deliverance

Parents and pitfalls

It's a . . .

HERE COMES ANOTHER CONTRACTION! OK, YOU'RE DOING FINE! BY THE WAY, HON, THAT CASSEROLE YOU MADE ME FOR TONIGHT. DO I HEAT THAT AT 350° OR 400°?
McPHERSON

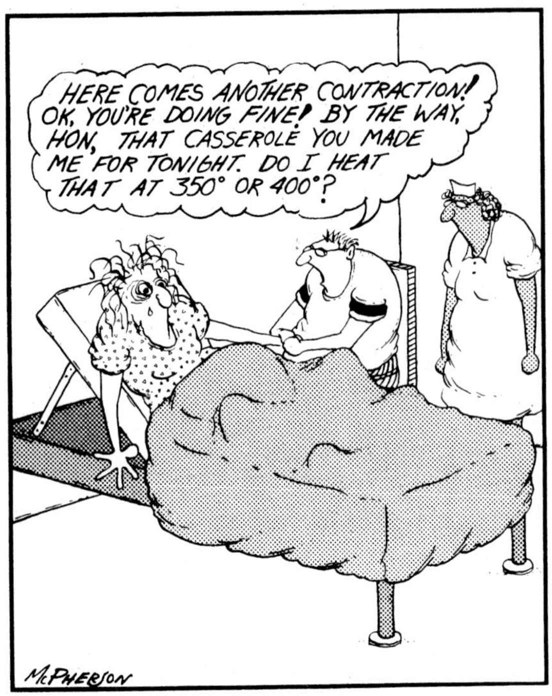

What not to say to your wife when she's in labor.

STRATTON

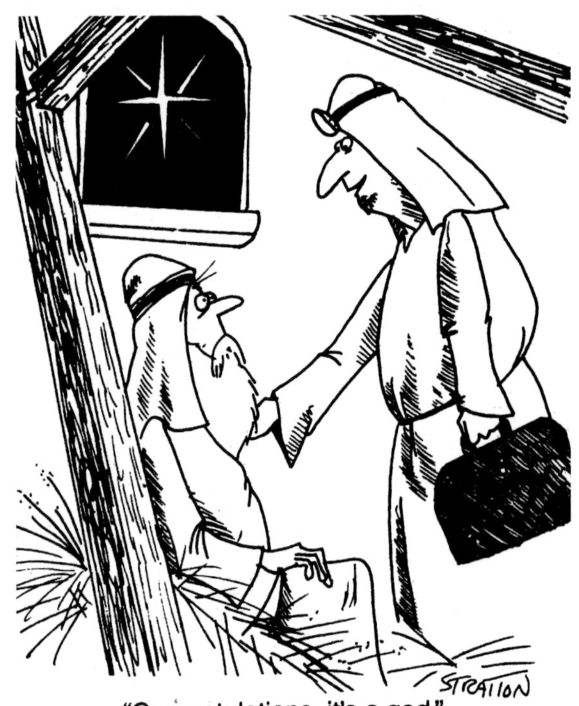

"Congratulations, it's a god."

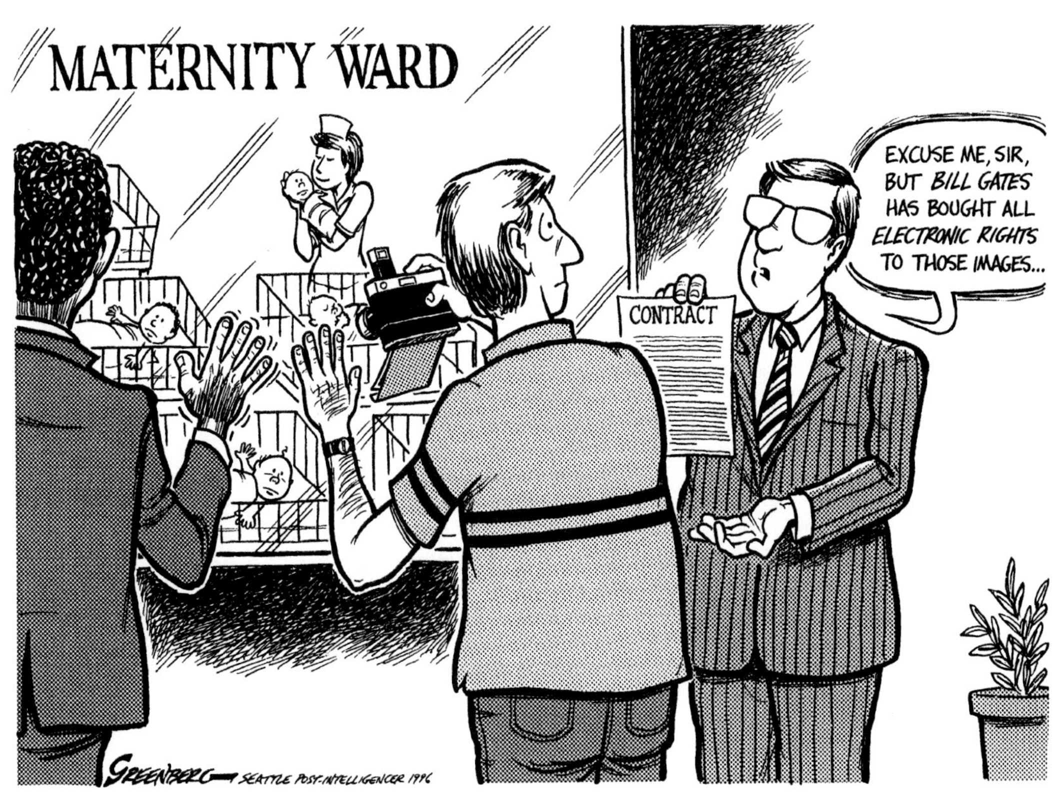
MATERNITY WARD
CONTRACT
EXCUSE ME, SIR, BUT BILL GATES HAS BOUGHT ALL ELECTRONIC RIGHTS TO THOSE IMAGES...
GREENBERG SEATTLE POST-INTELLIGENCER 1996

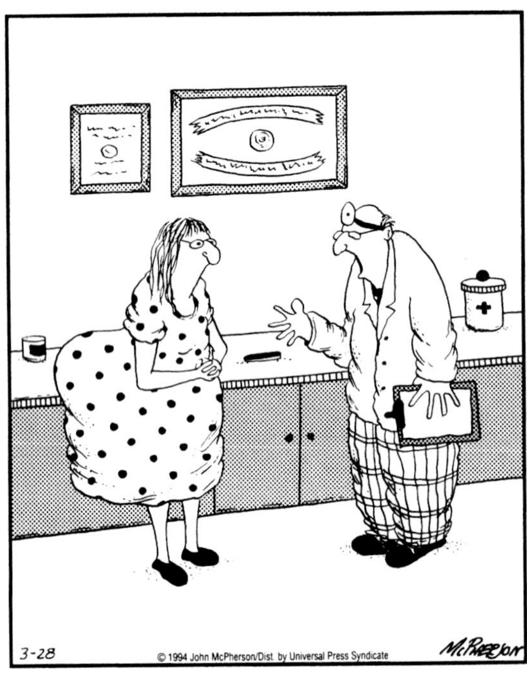

"Right now the baby is *not* in the proper position for delivery, but I'm confident it will shift in time for your due date."

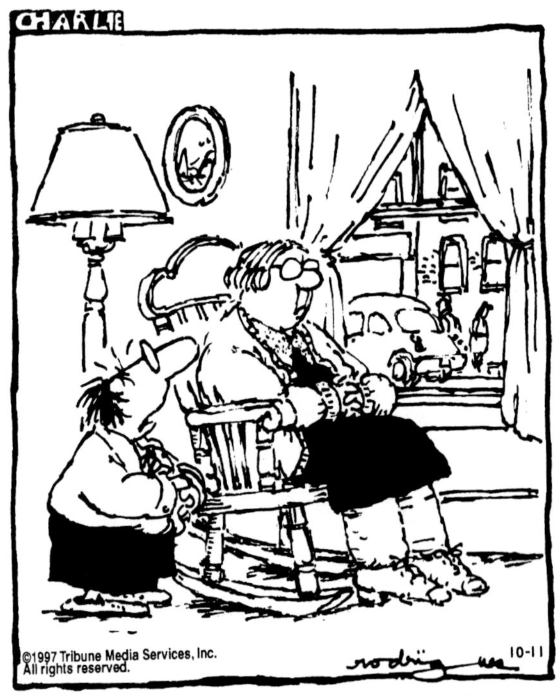

"Gee, Ma, I've apologized a hundred times. How long are you gonna be mad at me for bein' a breech baby?"

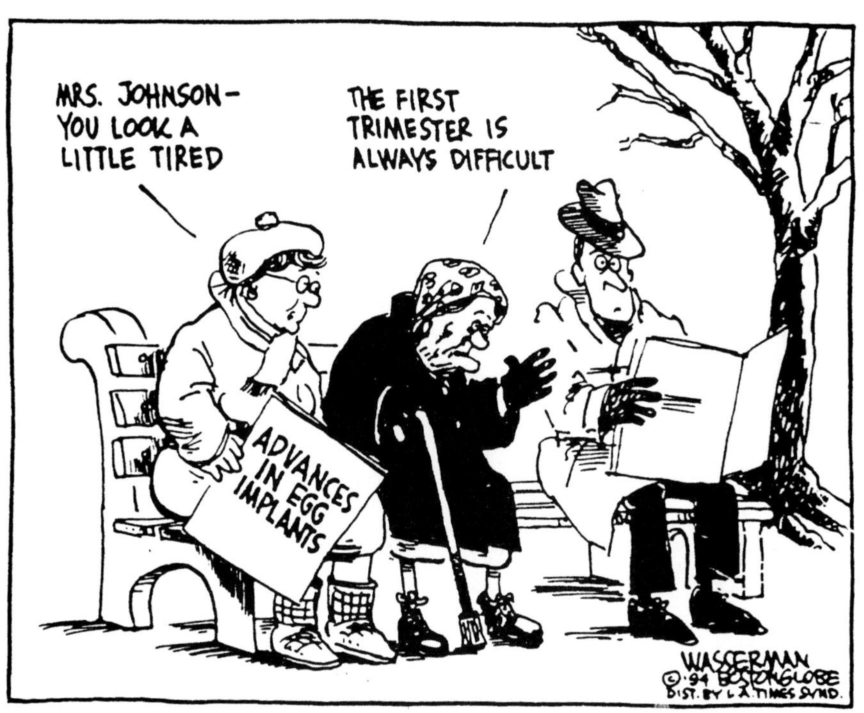

MRS. JOHNSON-
YOU LOOK A
LITTLE TIRED
THE FIRST
TRIMESTER IS
ALWAYS DIFFICULT
ADVANCES
IN EGG
IMPLANTS
WASSERMAN
©'94 BOSTON GLOBE
DIST. BY L.A. TIMES SYND.

HERMAN®

MATERNITY
Unger
7-30
© 1982 Jim Unger

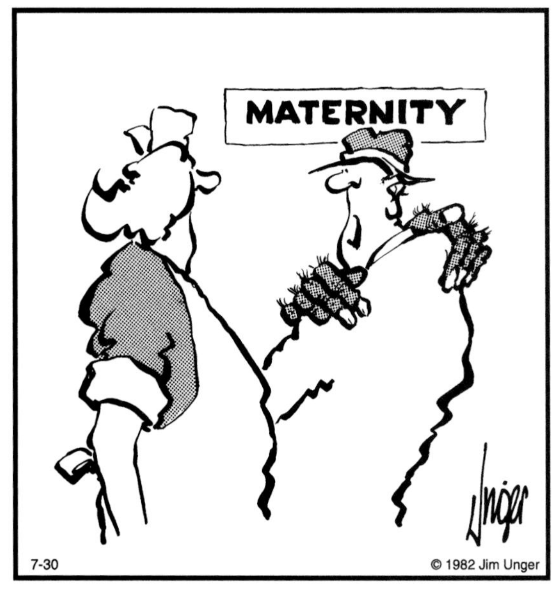

"You're absolutely certain this one's mine?"

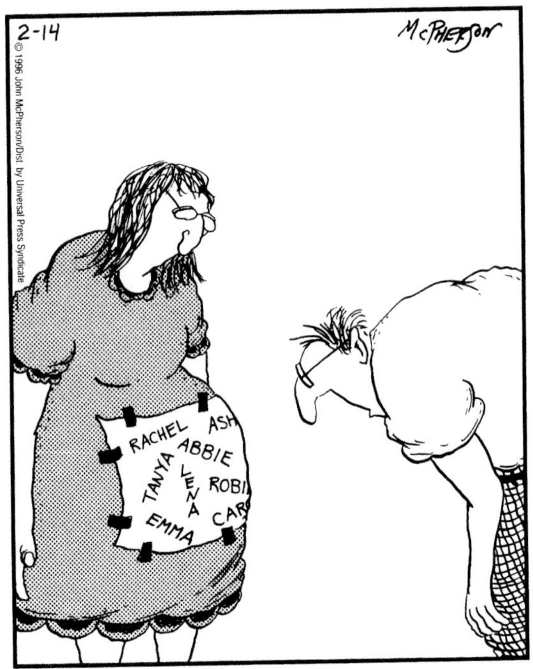

"OK, hold perfectly still! We go with whatever name the baby kicks at!"

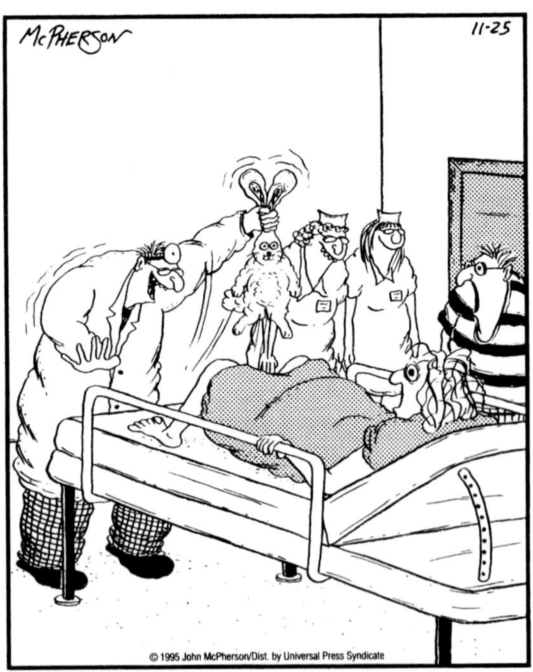

An amateur magician as well as an obstetrician, Dr. Kingsley felt it was important to bring some humor into the delivery room.

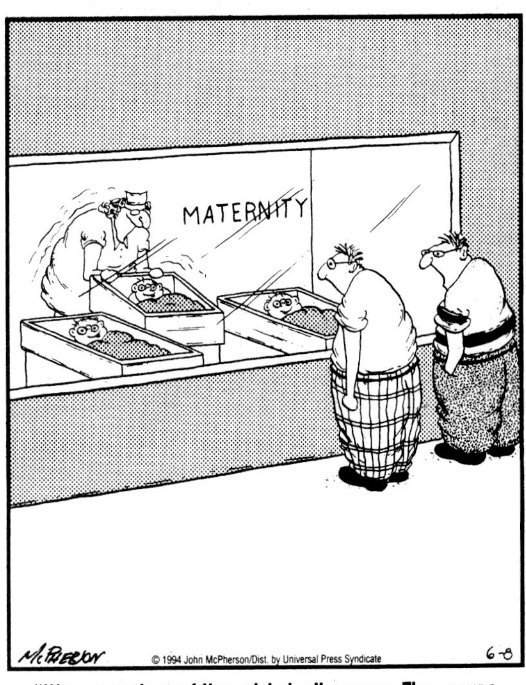

"It's a version of the old shell game. The nurse shuffles the babies around and you bet on which one is yours. So far I've lost 40 bucks."

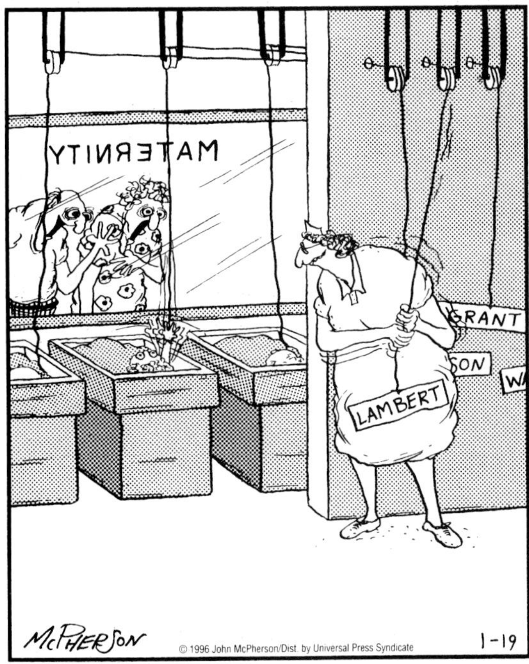

Thanks to some virtually invisible fishing line, Nurse Kretchner was able to evoke some priceless facial expressions from proud parents and grandparents.

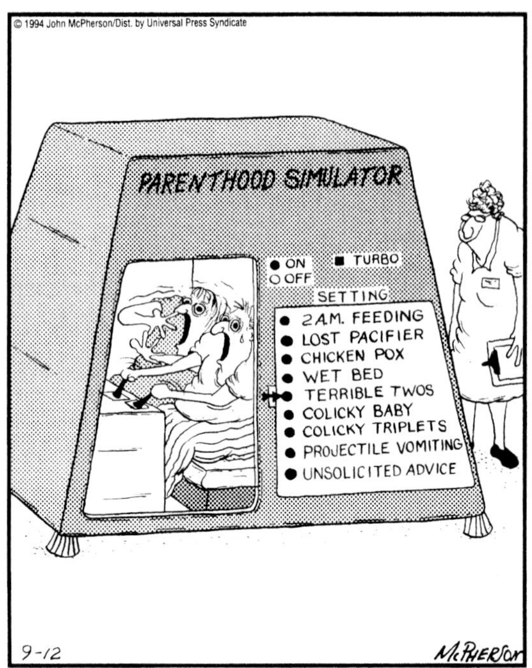

In an effort to prepare expectant parents for the challenges that lie ahead, many obstetricians' offices have installed parenthood simulators.

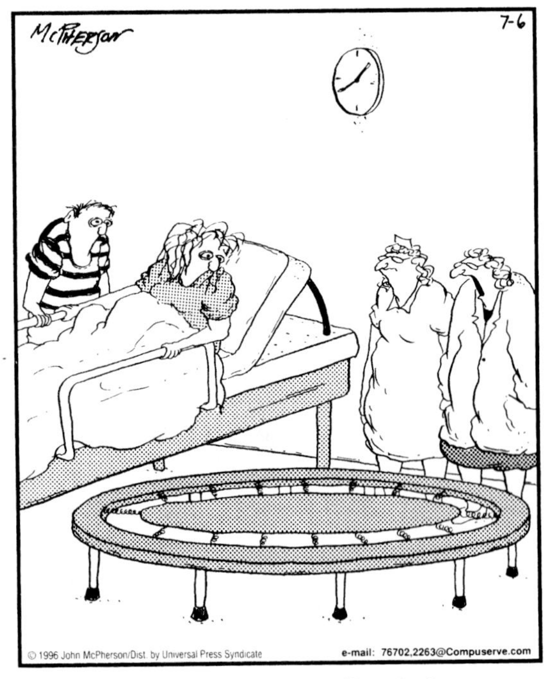

"We like to try all our options before using drugs to induce labor."

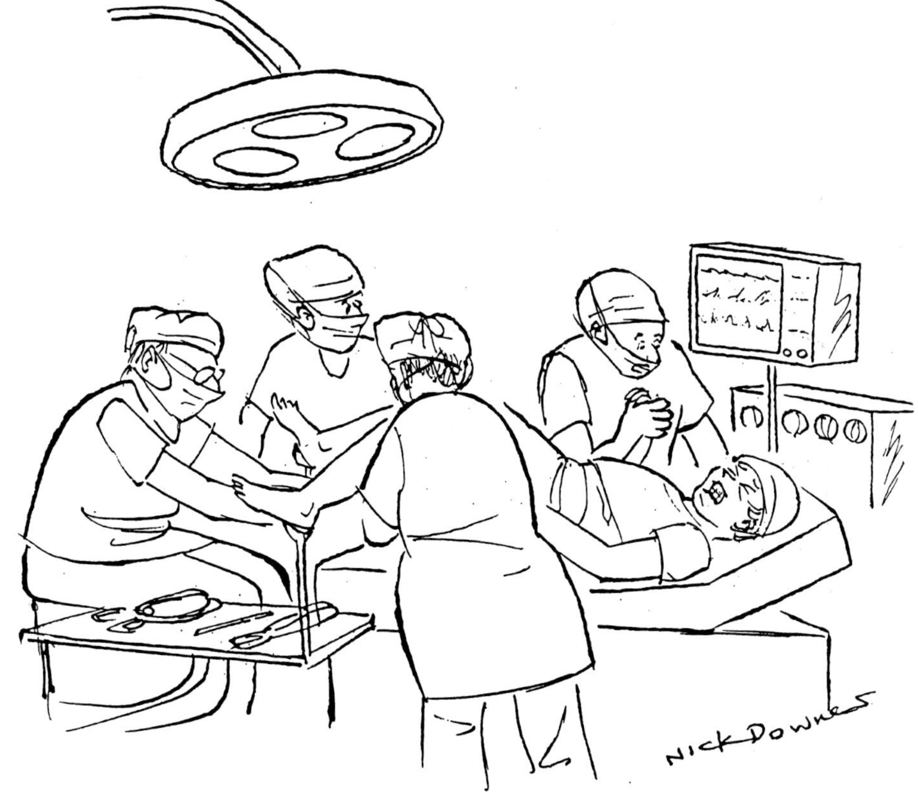

"Push, Dear! The child will be late for pre-school!"

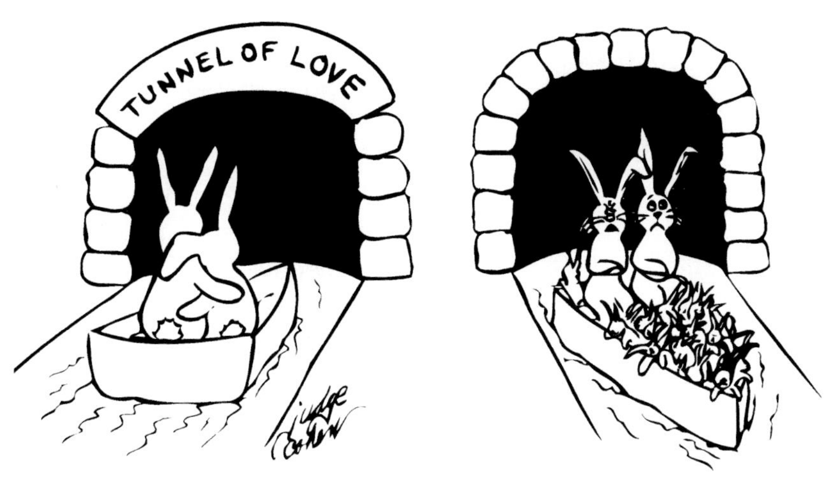

"That's it, Clyde! You're getting a vasectomy."

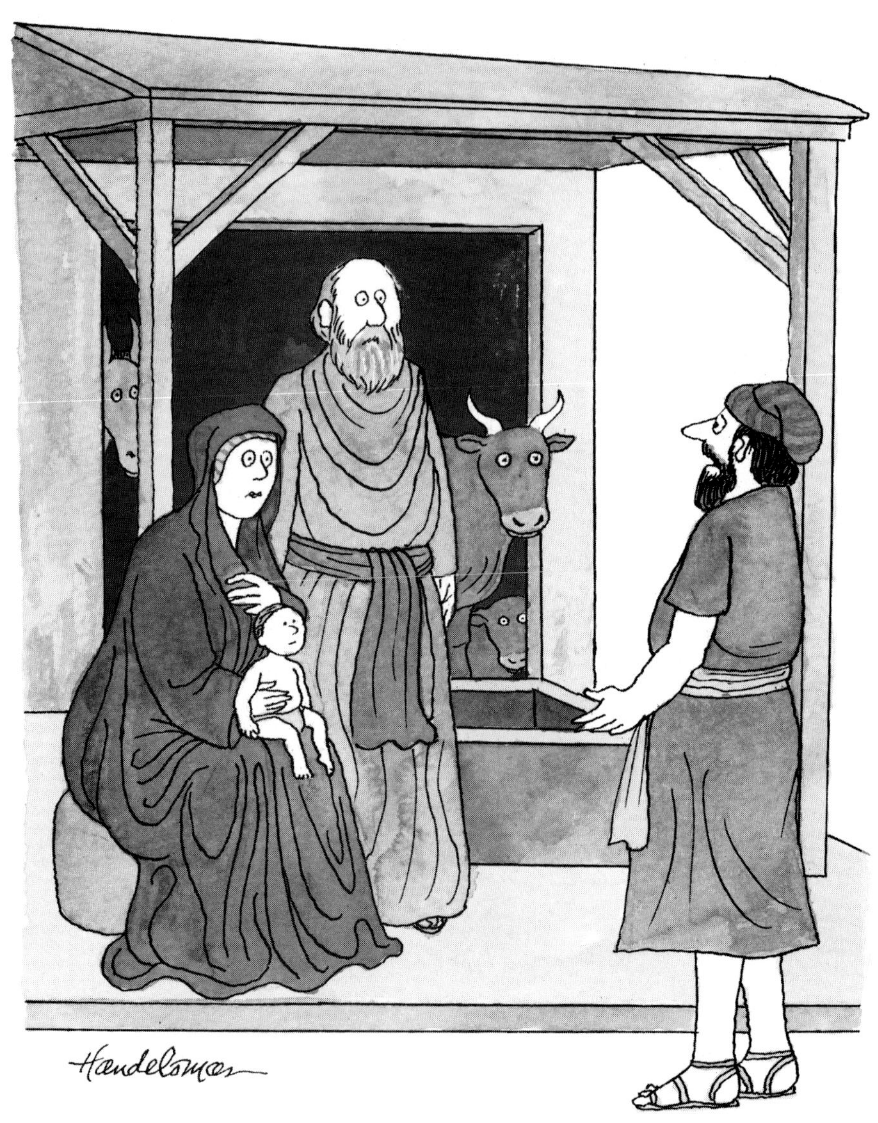

"Sorry, folks, but your insurance doesn't cover more than one day in the manger."

11. Help! It's an Emergency

I need help now!

Something's wrong

Hurry up!

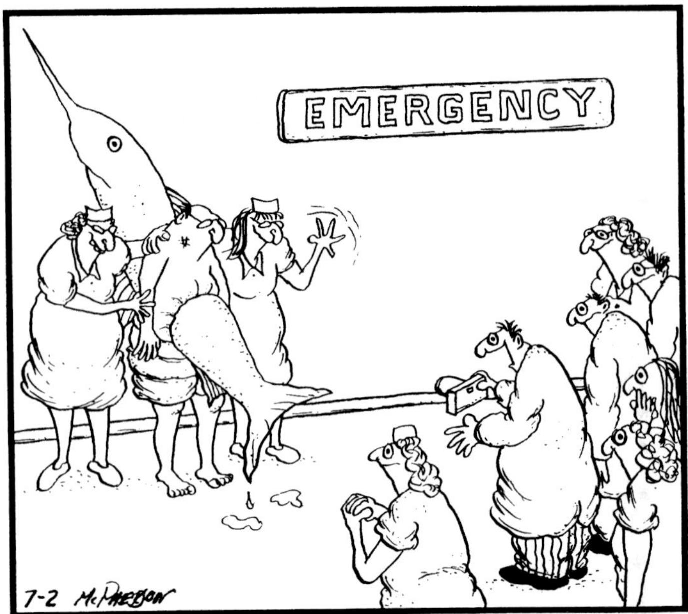

"If you don't mind, Mr. Morris, I'd like to get one more photo with you, me and some of the ambulance attendants, and then we'll get you right over to X-ray."

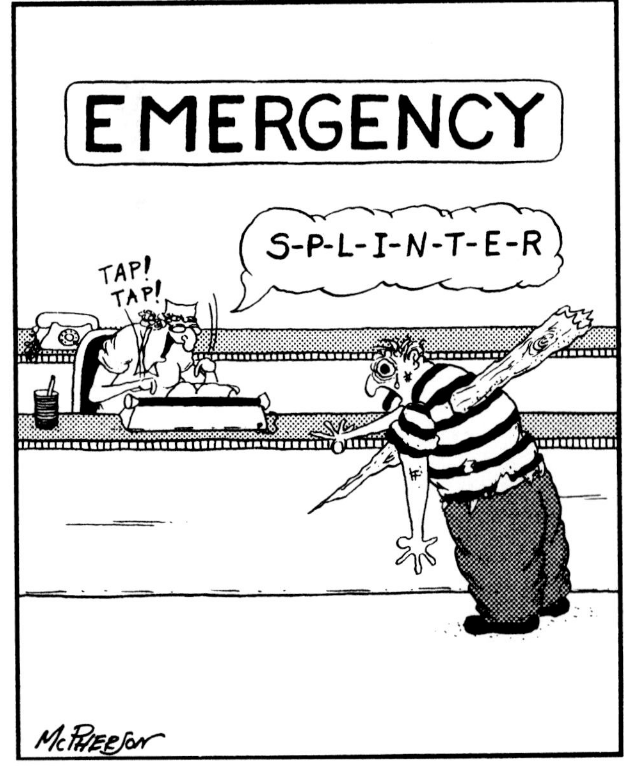

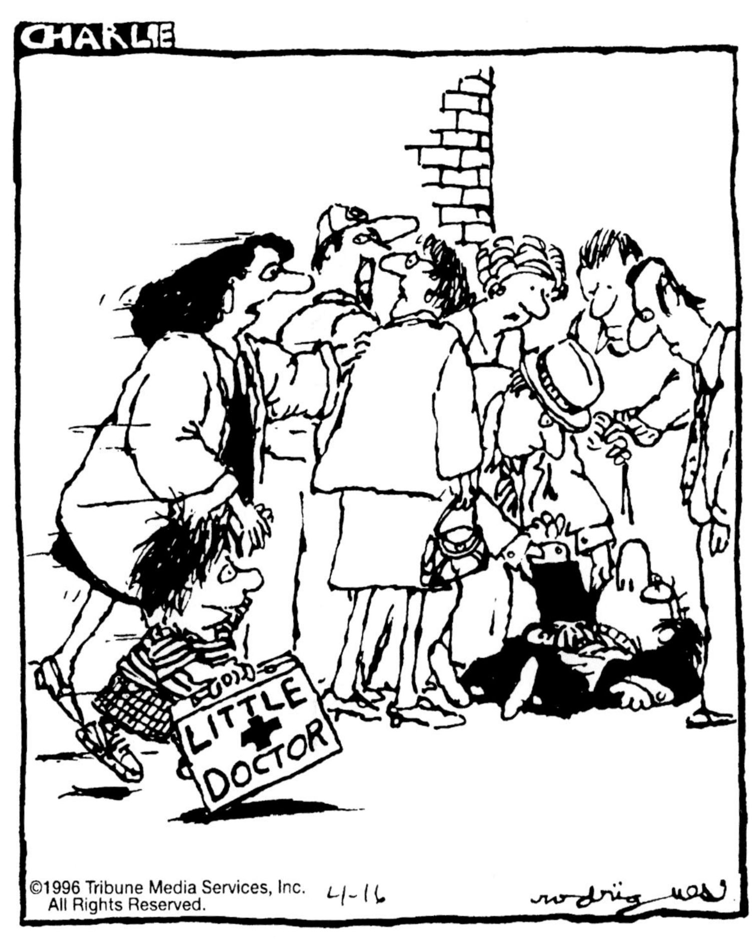

"Let me through, my little boy wants to play doctor!"

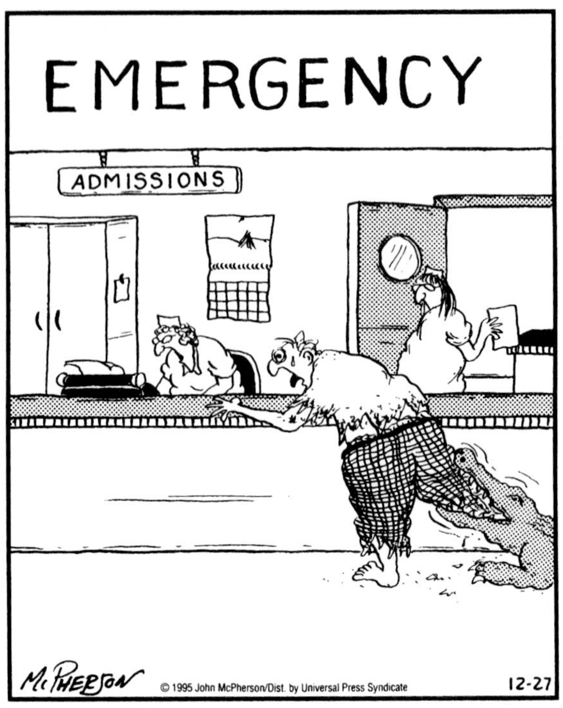

"Oh, shoot! Donna, could you run up to supply on the eighth floor and get me some correction tape?"

HERMAN®

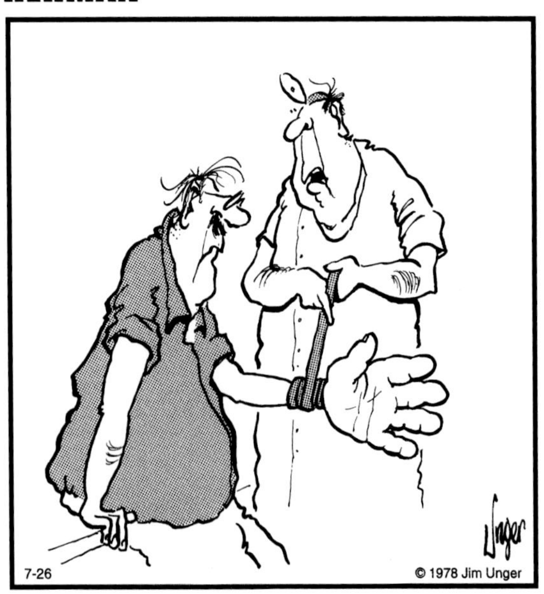

"That too tight?"

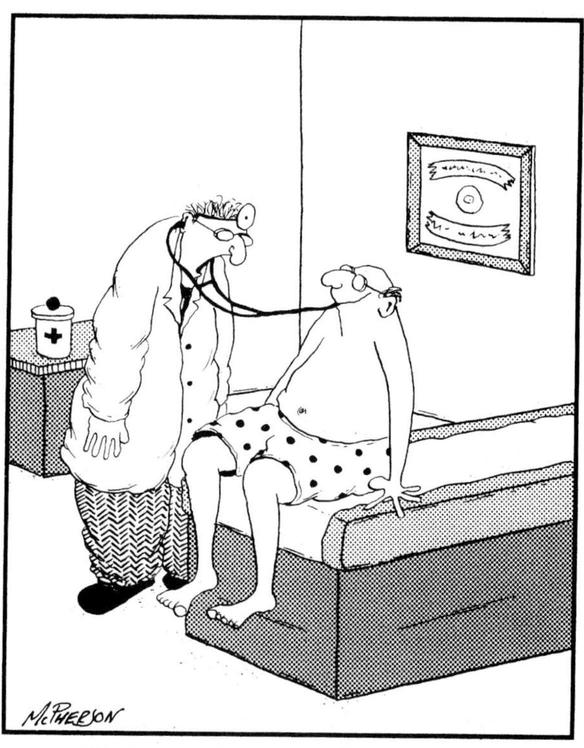

"Mr. Farnsley, I haven't got the slightest idea what song you're humming. Please take the stethoscope out of your mouth so we can finish your examination."

HERMAN®

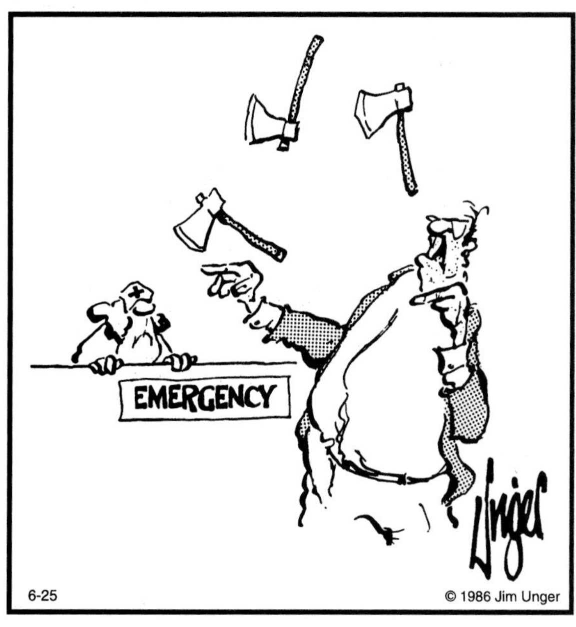

"I can't stop."

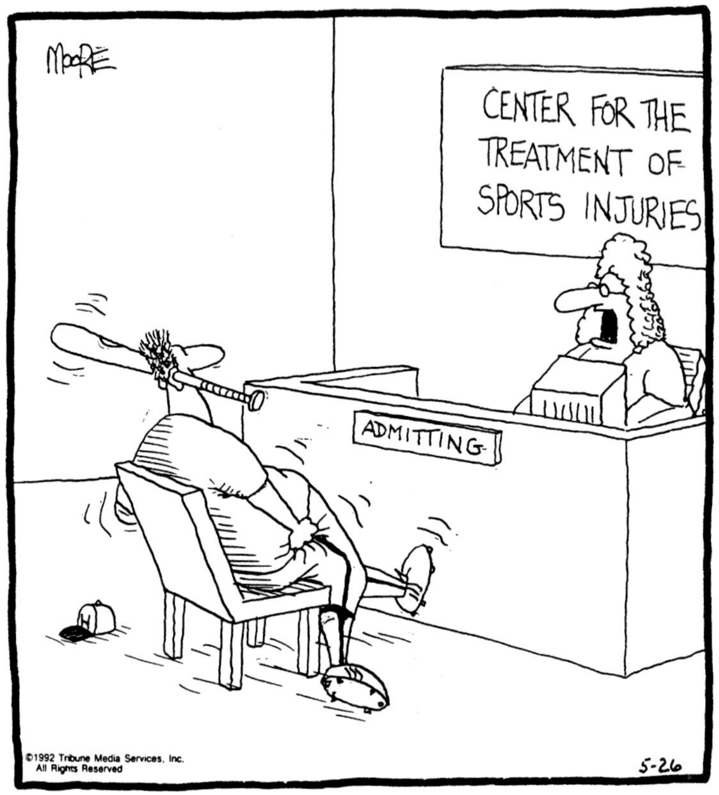

" ... Stop squirming, Mr. Silcox. The sooner we fill out these forms, the sooner we'll find out exactly what it is that's wrong with you."

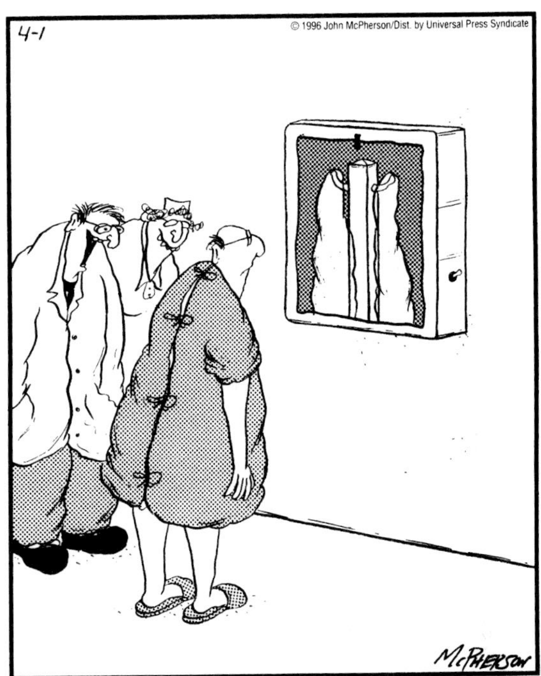

"We were pretty worried about you until we discovered that the power on the X-ray machine was set way too high and we had actually gotten an image of a coat rack in the room behind you."

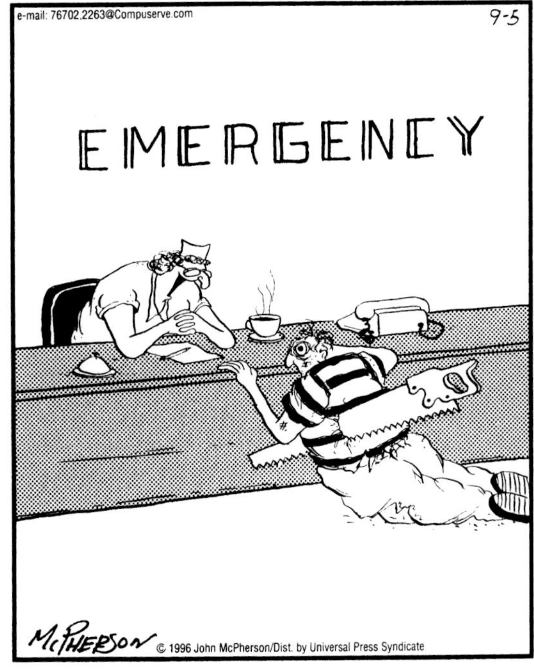

"I'm sorry, sir, but your insurance company requires that you first get a referral slip from your primary care physician before we can treat you."

REAL LIFE ADVENTURES by Gary Wise and Lance Aldrich

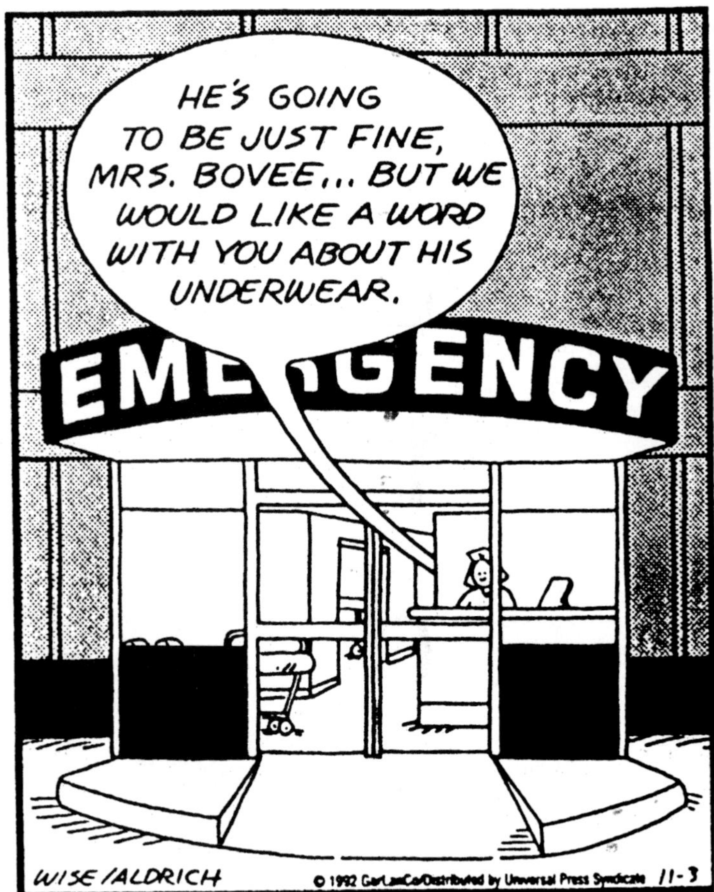

Your mother's worst nightmare.

12.

Cosmetic Encounters of the Third Kind

Getting under your skin

Face off

Adventures in the skin trade

Rash decisions

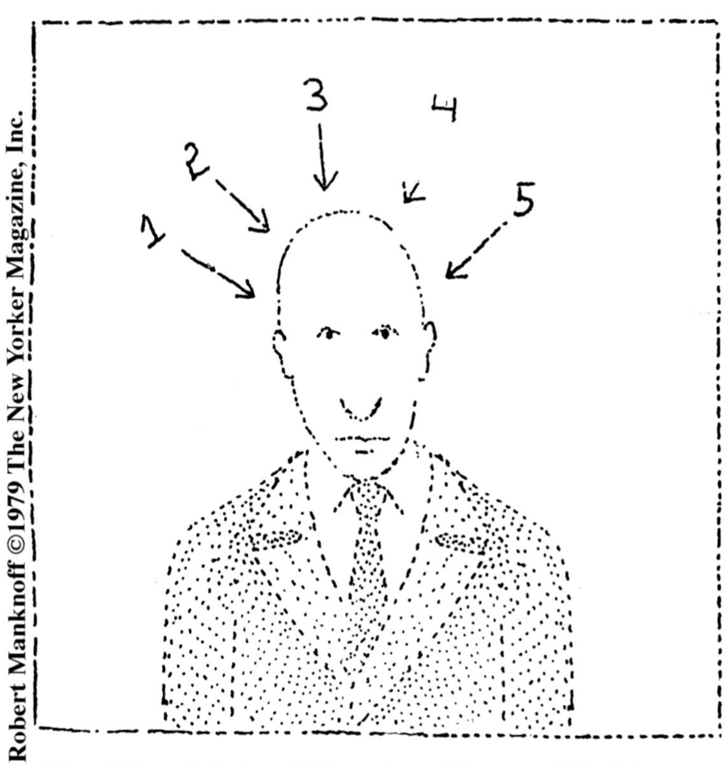

The Five Major Warning Signs of Baldness

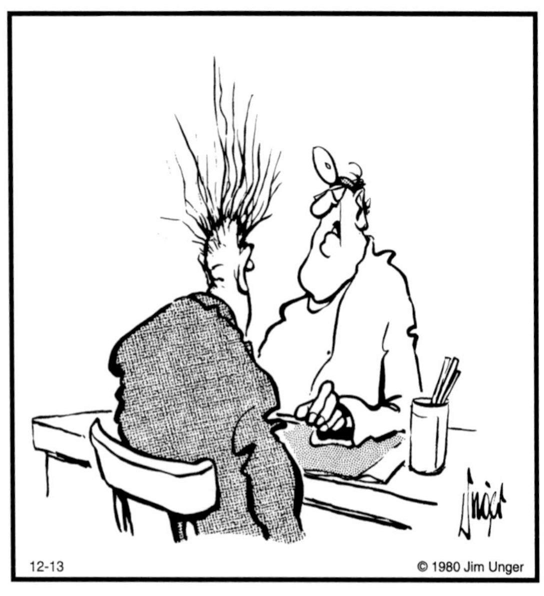

"Your head's rejecting your hair transplant!"

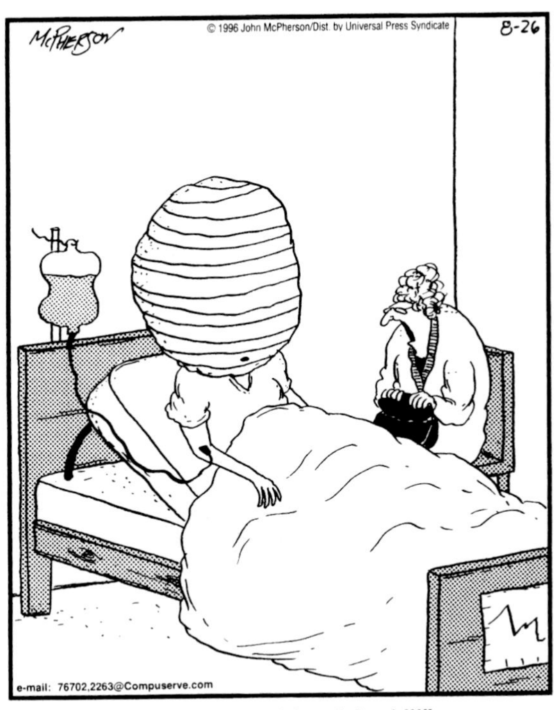

"I *told* you not to pick at it!"

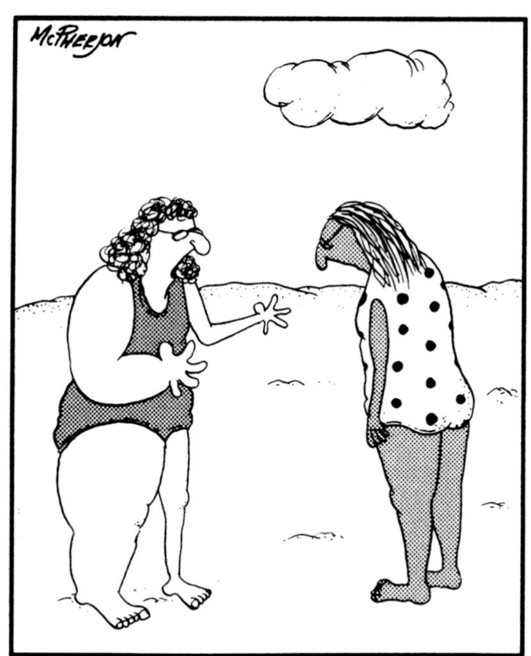

"So, to make a long story short, the insurance company tells us in the midst of it all that it'll pay for only half of the liposuction."

Farcus

by David Waisglass
Gordon Coulthart

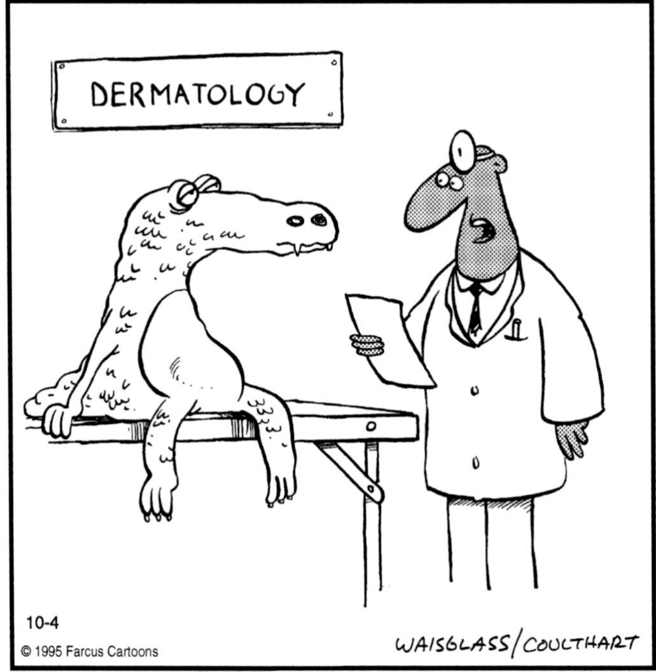

"I can prescribe moisturizers, but you'd still make a terrific handbag."

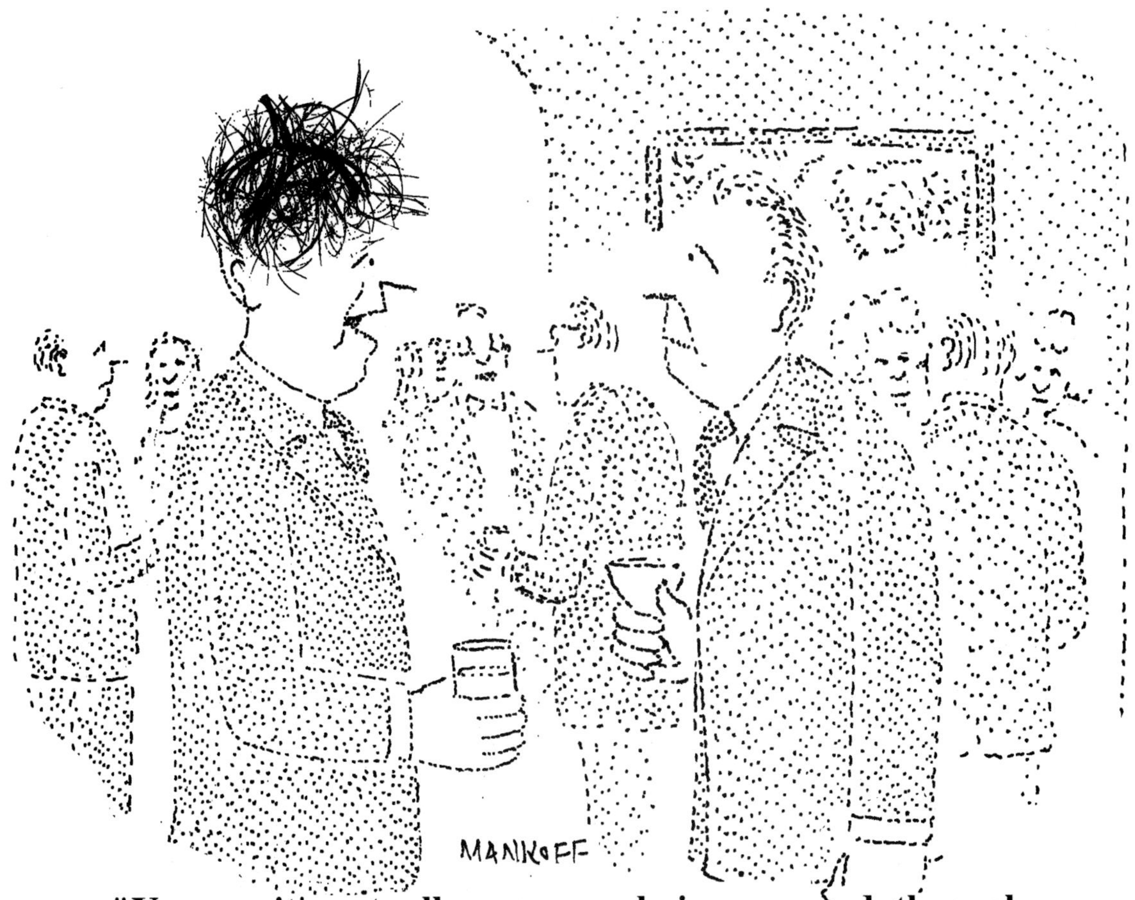

"You see, it's actually your own hair recovered, through painstaking research, from past visits to the barber, and then pasted back on your head."

HERMAN®

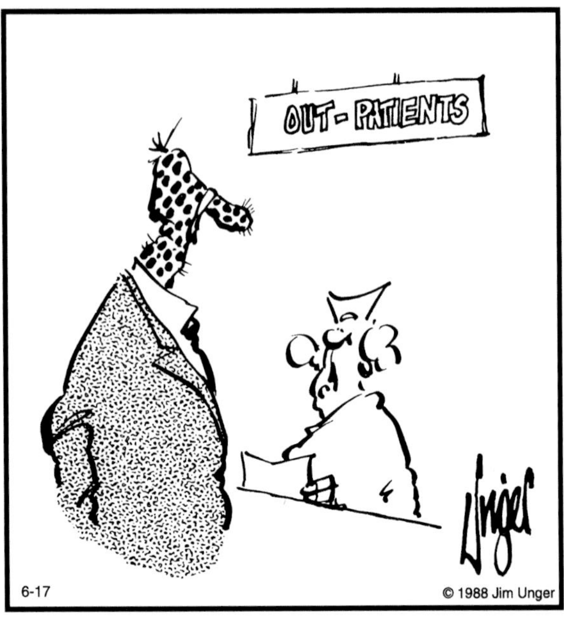

"Do you want Dr. Watson, the skin specialist or Dr. Watson, the gynecologist?"

HERMAN®

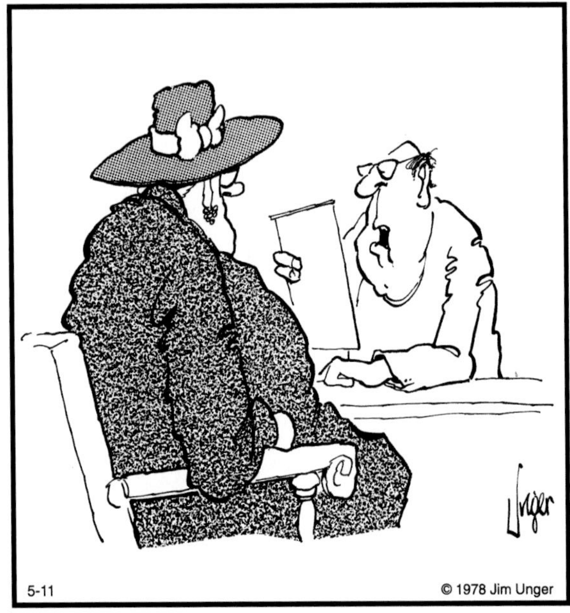

"Forget the facelift. I think we'll try lowering your body."

IN THE BLEACHERS By Steve Moore

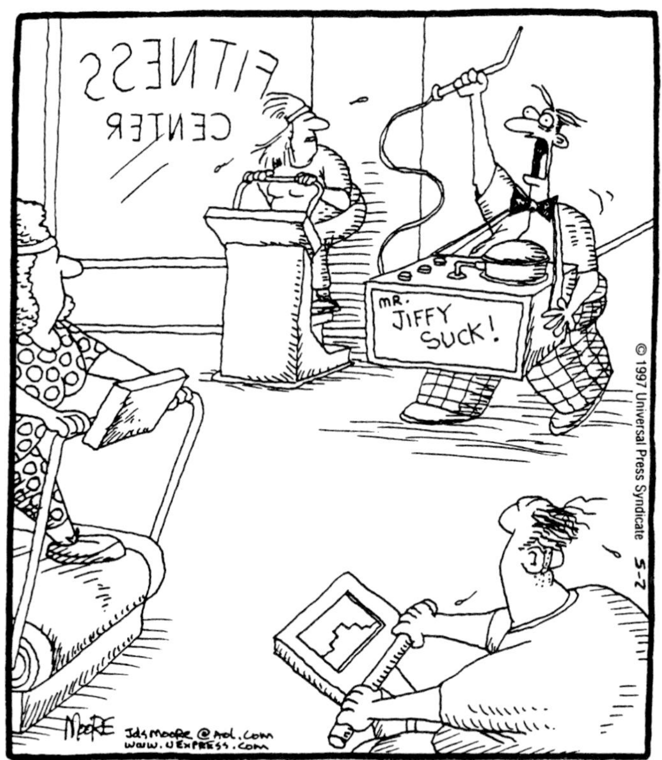

"Liposuction! Liposuction! Yo, liposuction!"

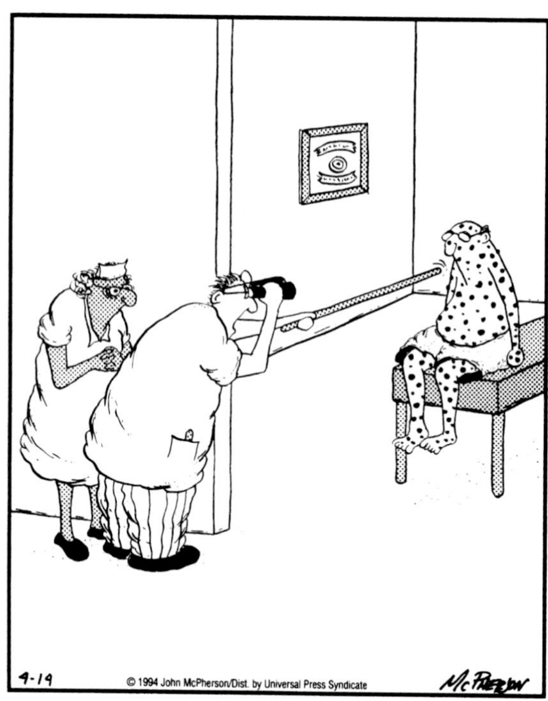

"Stick the other end of this in your mouth and say 'Ahh.'"

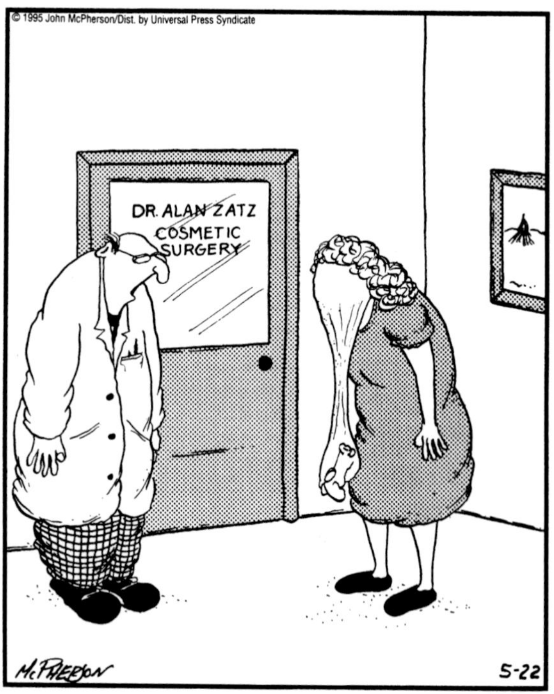

"Unfortunately, Carolyn, your body has rejected your face lift."

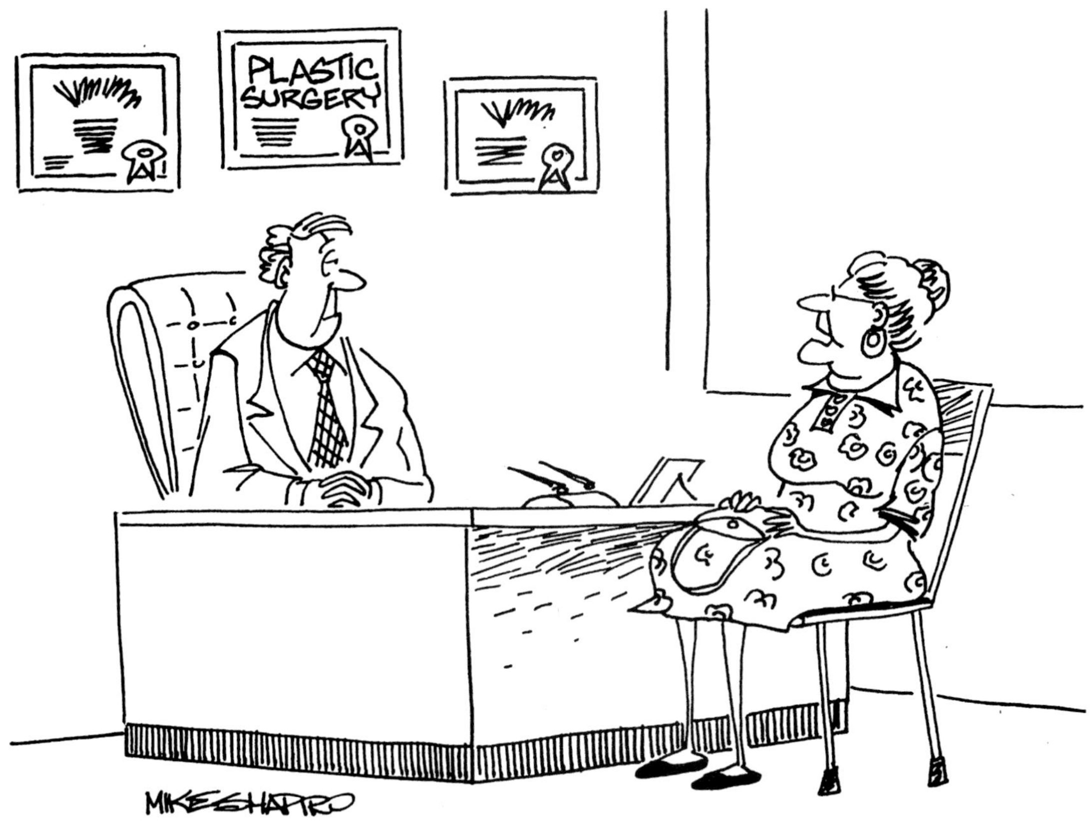

"I want to look like Cindy Crawford."

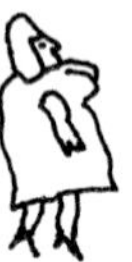

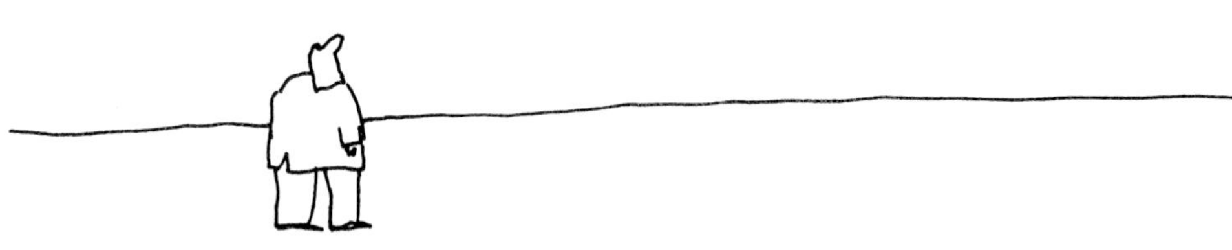

RICHARD'S LONELINESS ONLY DEEPENED AFTER SYLVIA'S HELIUM BREAST IMPLANTS.

CALLAHAN

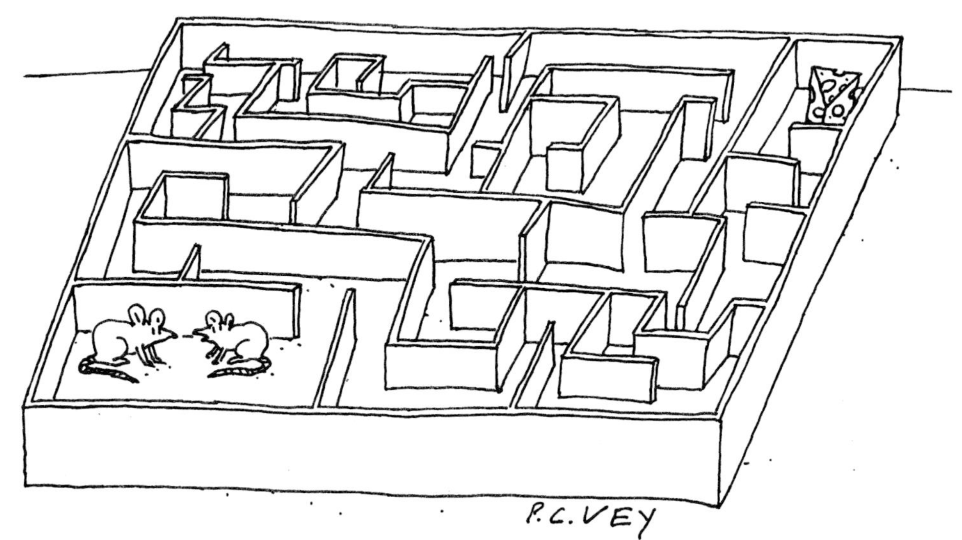

"My doctor tells me to stay away from dairy products."

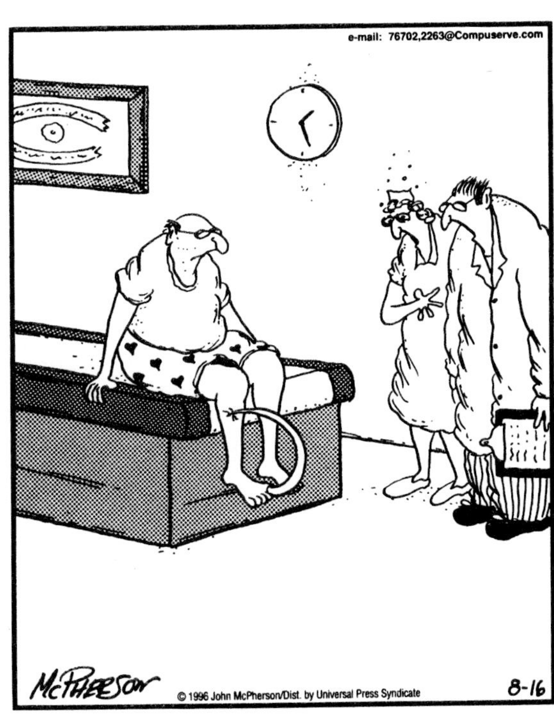

"Now *that*, Mr. Fillman, is what I call an ingrown toenail!"

MISTER BOFFO

by Joe Martin

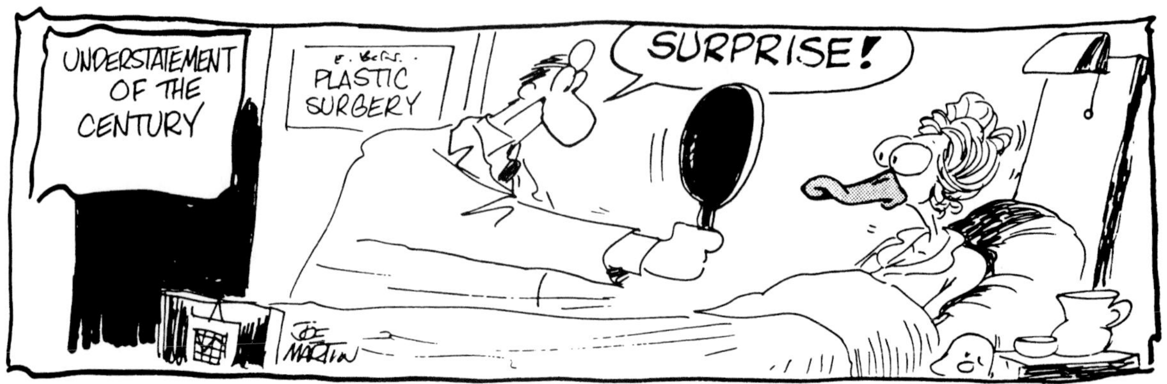

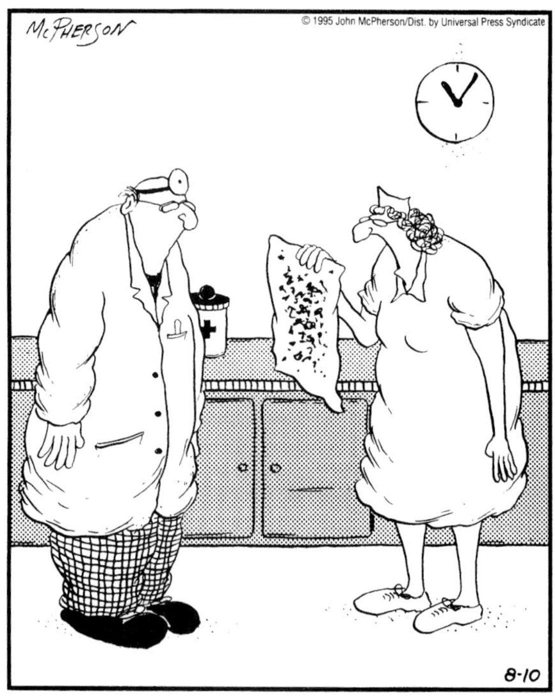

"Mrs. Nortman just sent in this fax of a rash that she's got on her stomach."

13.

Funny Bone

Orthopedic humor

Fractures and farces

Breaks me up

Farcus

by David Waisglass
Gordon Coulthart

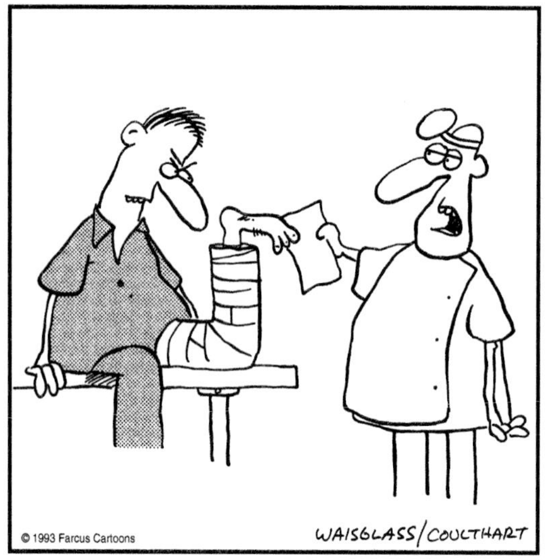

"That's *Dr.* Idiot to you!"

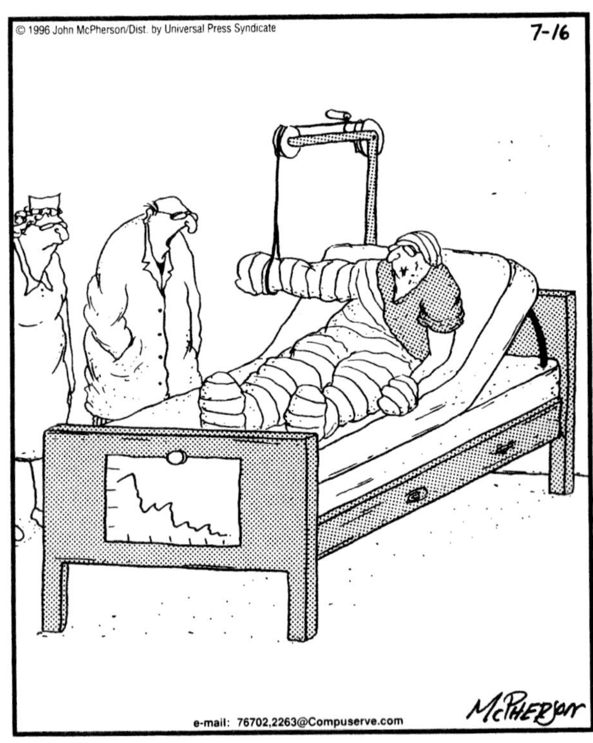

"Your insurance company is refusing to pay your medical bills due to a pre-existing condition. It says you were already an idiot before you decided to Rollerblade down the interstate."

IN THE BLEACHERS By Steve Moore

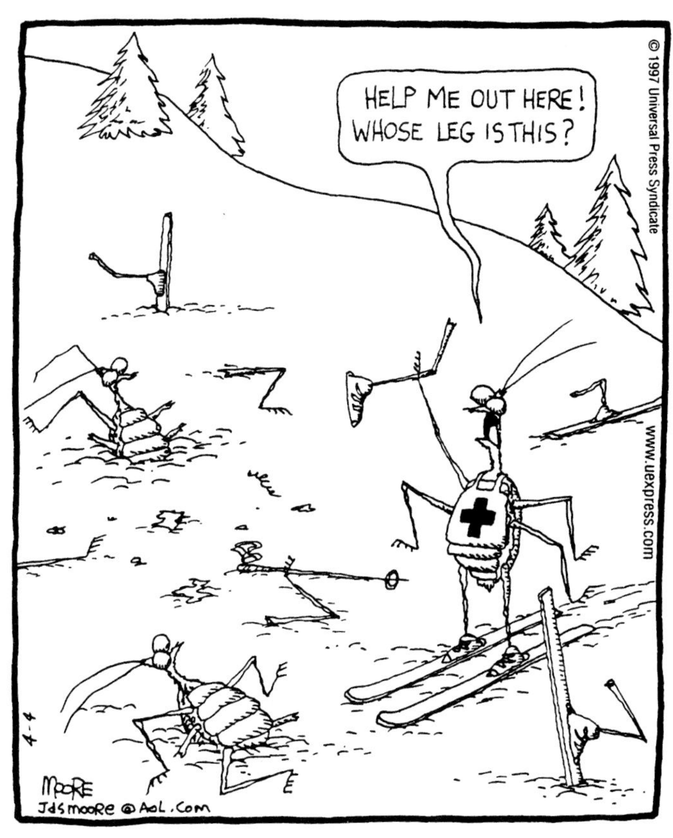

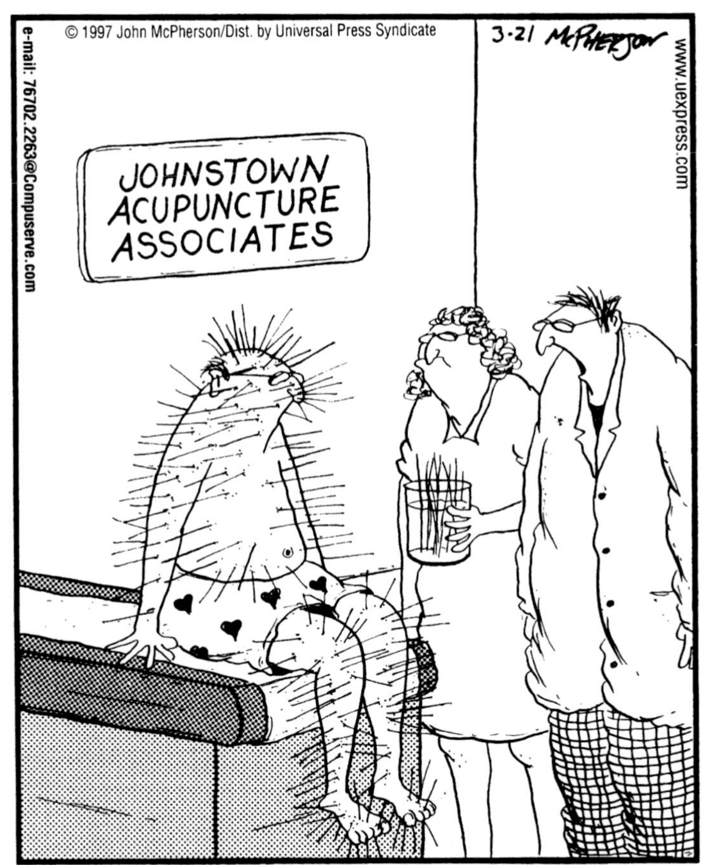

"You gotta be kidding! Your back *still* hurts?!"

MISTER BOFFO

by Joe Martin

THE ABSOLUTE LAST THING YOU WANT TO HEAR FROM YOUR CHIROPRACTOR AT A TIME LIKE THIS
I FELT SOMETHING POP!?

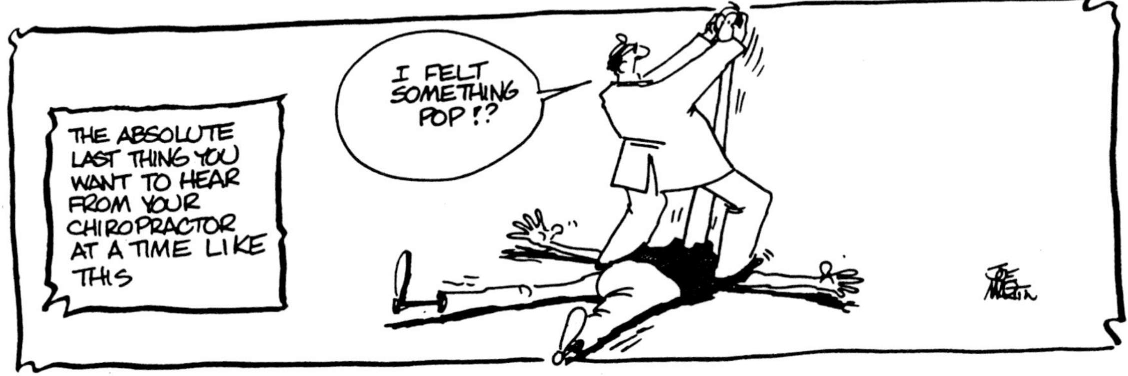

IN THE BLEACHERS

By Steve Moore

E-MAIL, SCHMEE-MAIL: JDSMOORE @AOL.COM
MOORE
© 1996 Universal Press Syndicate
2-17

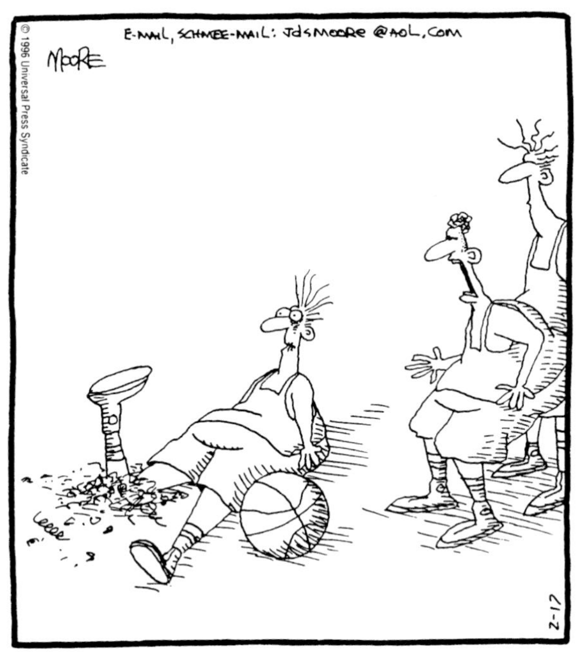

"Where do you hurt? Your back? Ankle? Shoulder? Neck? Knee? ... He blinked! I think it's his knee."

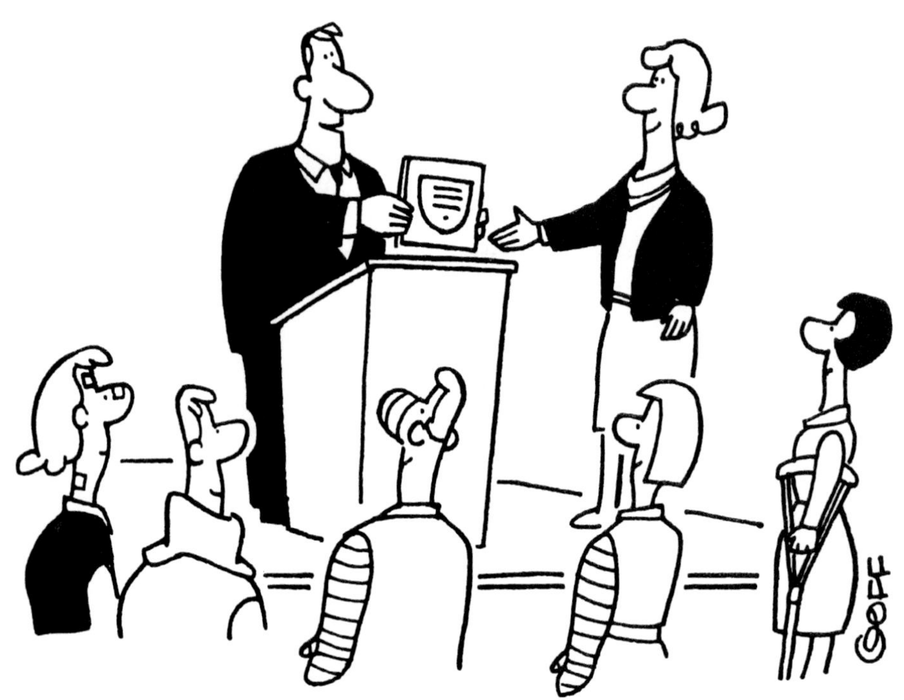

"The winner of this year's safe-driving award is Judy Martinez!"

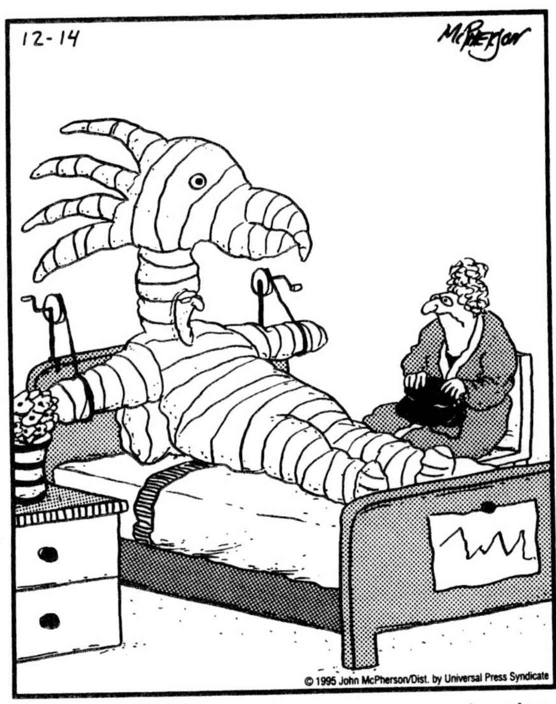

"The intern who worked on me was an art major before going to med school."

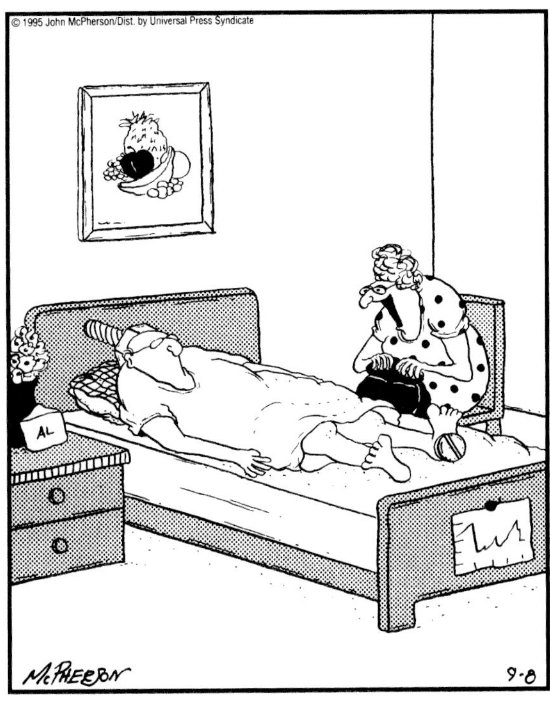

"The doctor says the pin can come out in three months."

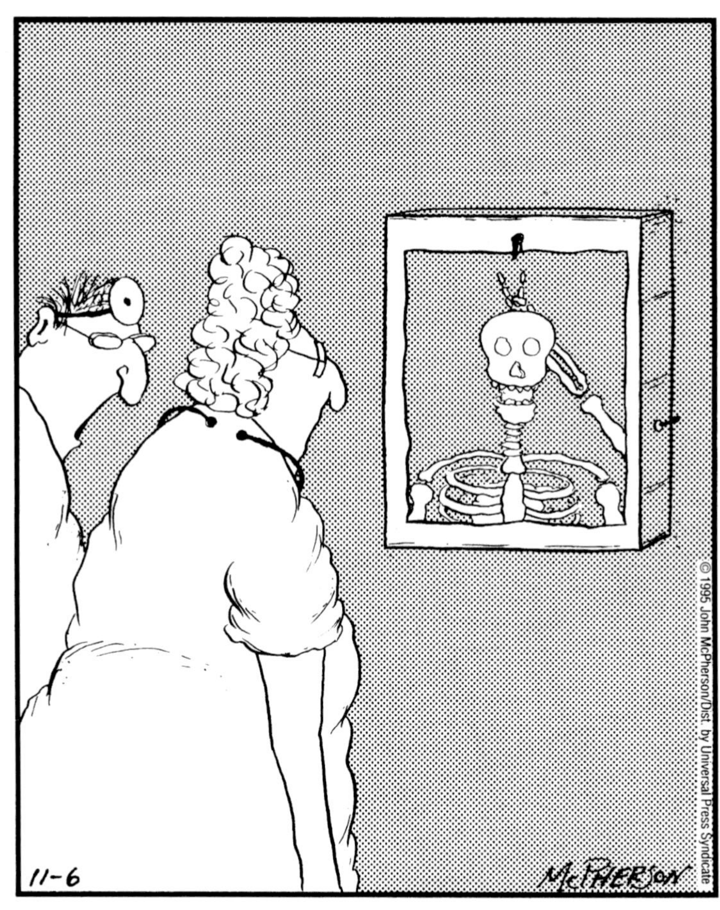

"Who's the wiseguy down in X-ray?"

14.

Weight and See

Shedding pounds

Lifestyles for progress

The joke of cooking

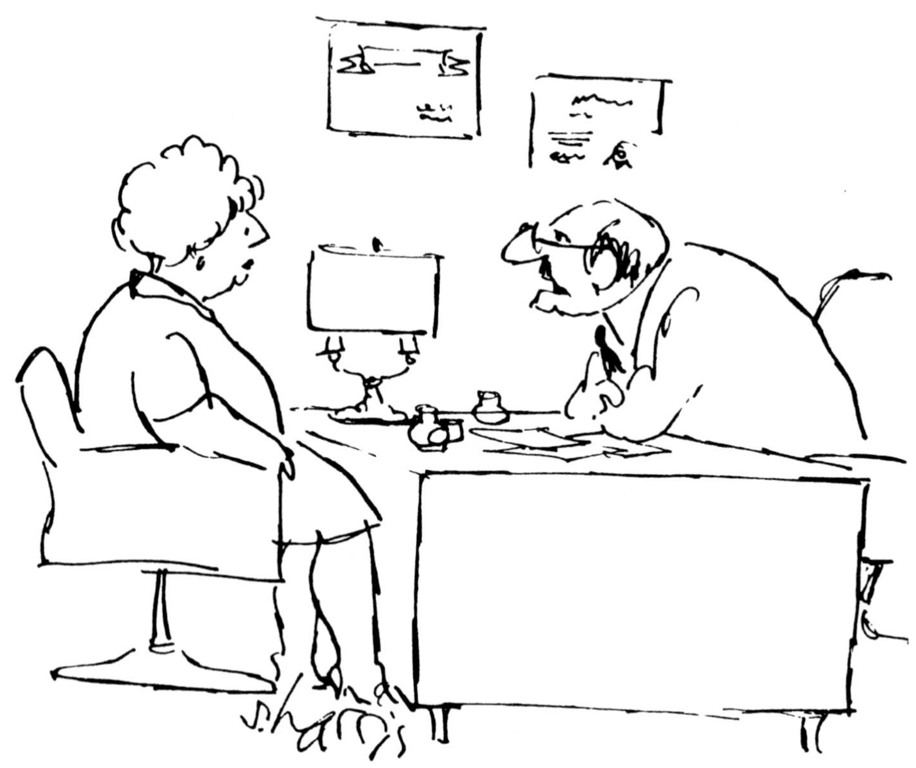

"It's partly glandular and partly 8,500 calories per day."

US & THEM

by Wiley Miller & Susan Dewar

WELCOME TO THE BETTY FORD CLINIC, MR. PYLE... WHAT IS THE NATURE OF YOUR ADDICTION?
ICE CREAM
CHECK IN
UH-H-H, HUH.
I'M AFRAID WE JUST DON'T CONSIDER ICE CREAM AS AN ADDICTIVE SUBSTANCE
...IT'S BEN AND JERRY'S COCONUT ALMOND FUDGE CHUNK
CODE RED!!
WILEY ©1996 1-16

CHARLIE
3-11
©1997 Tribune Media Services, Inc.
All rights reserved.

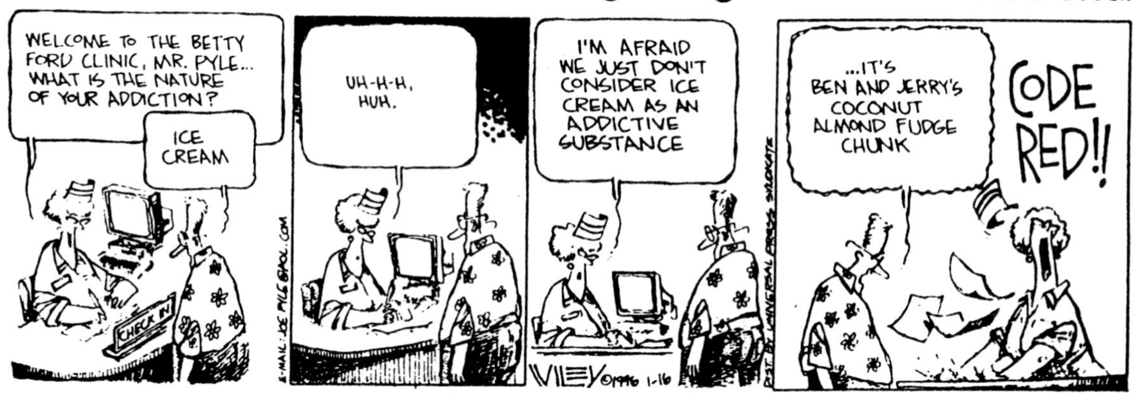

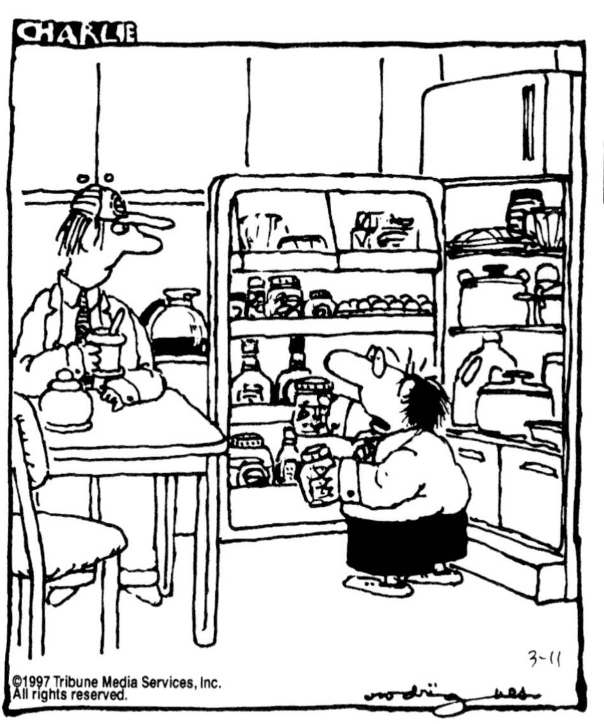

“My doctor put me on a strict diet.
I can only eat from my fridge door.”

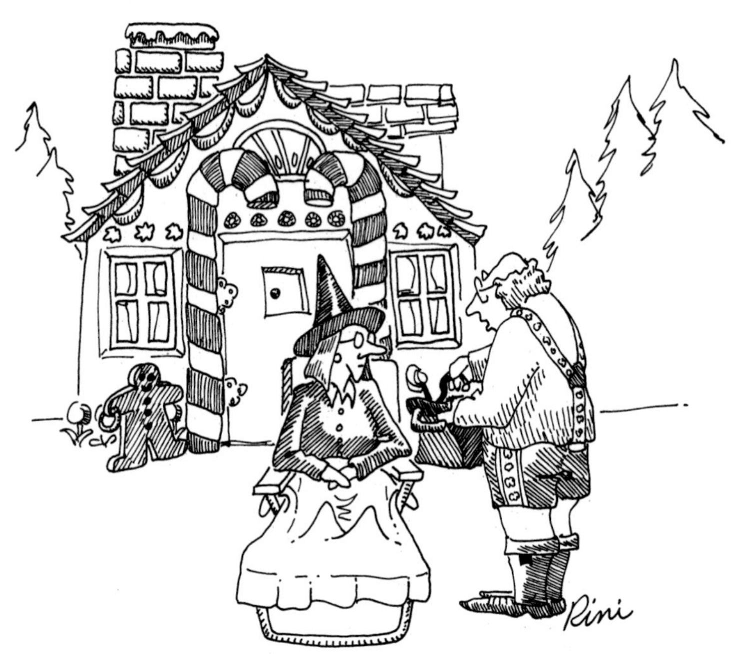

"With your cholesterol so high, I suggest switching your diet from little Bavarian children, to Southern Californians."

HERMAN®

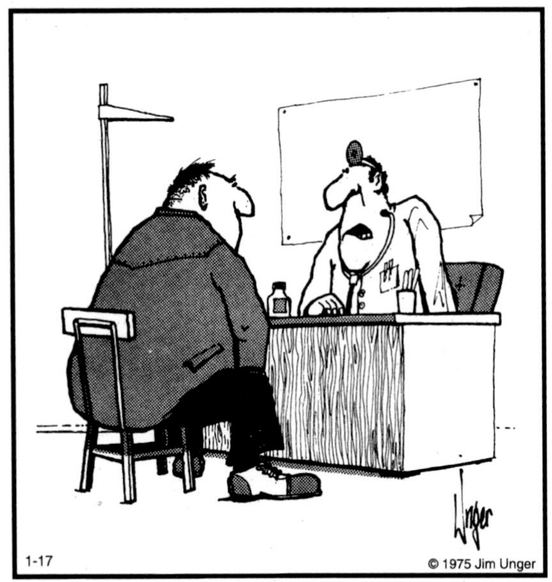

"Let me put it this way ... for your weight you should be thirty-seven feet tall."

Farcus

by David Waisglass
Gordon Coulthart

1-4
© 1997 Farcus Cartoons
WAISGLASS/COULTHART
www.farcus.com

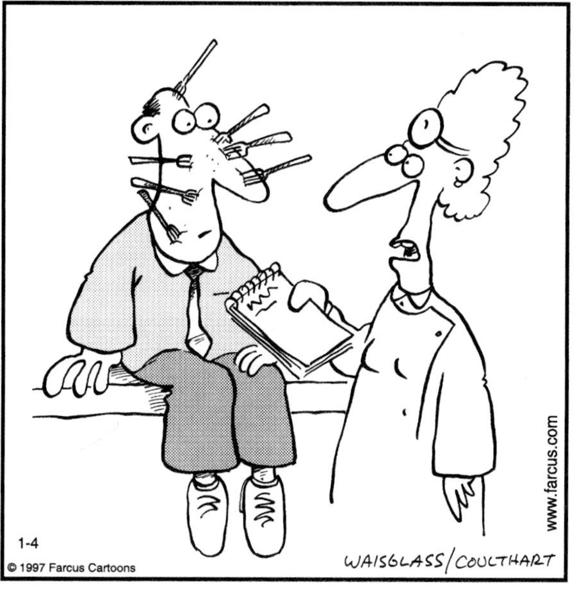

"I'm afraid, Mr. Johnson, you have an eating disorder."

Mom probably wouldn't buy us one, but you have to learn to make your own choices, Dad.
ICE CREAM
SIPRESS

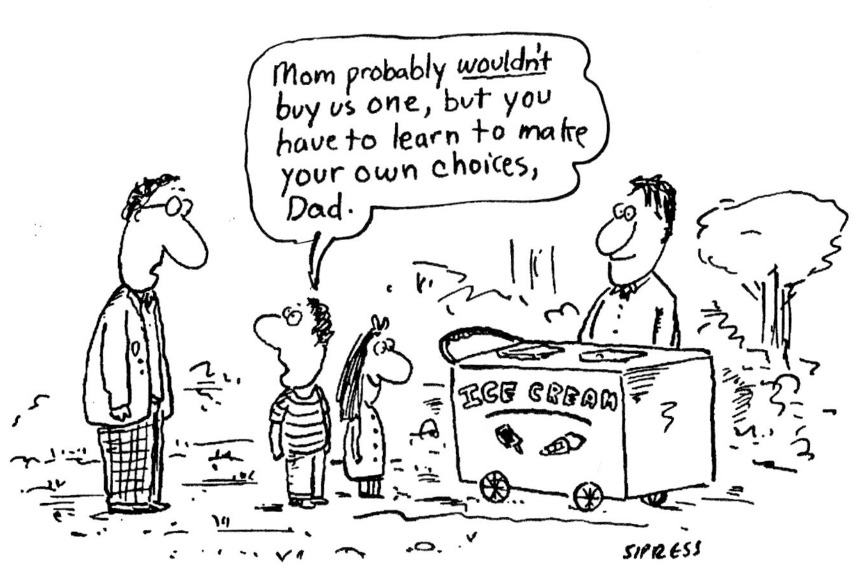

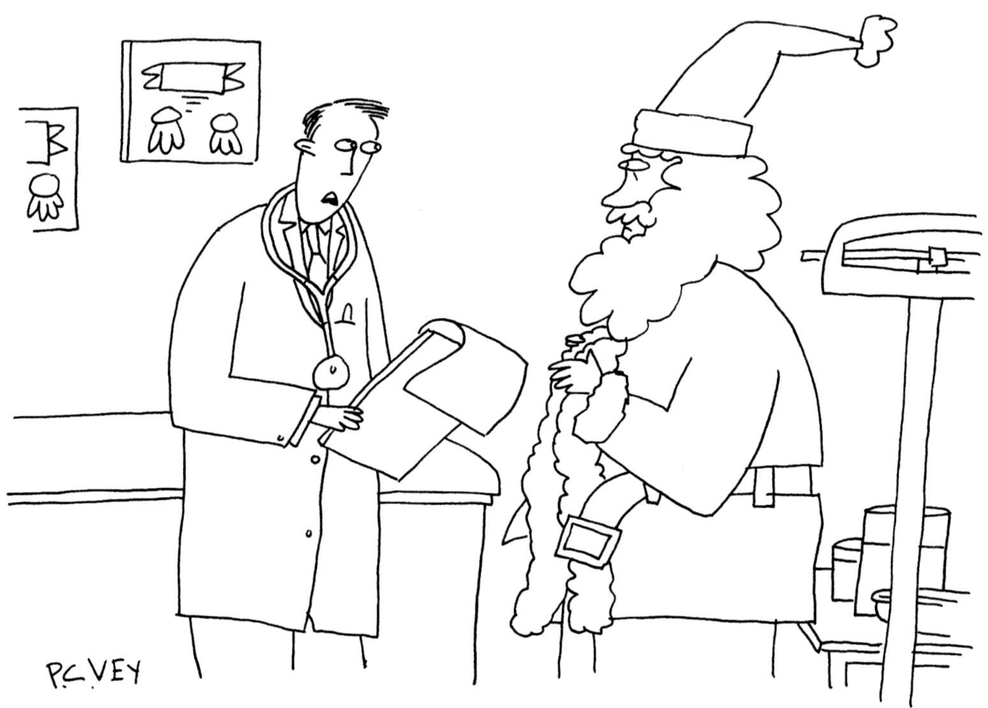

". . . and since you're a lactose intolerant borderline diabetic I think you should cut out the milk and cookies."

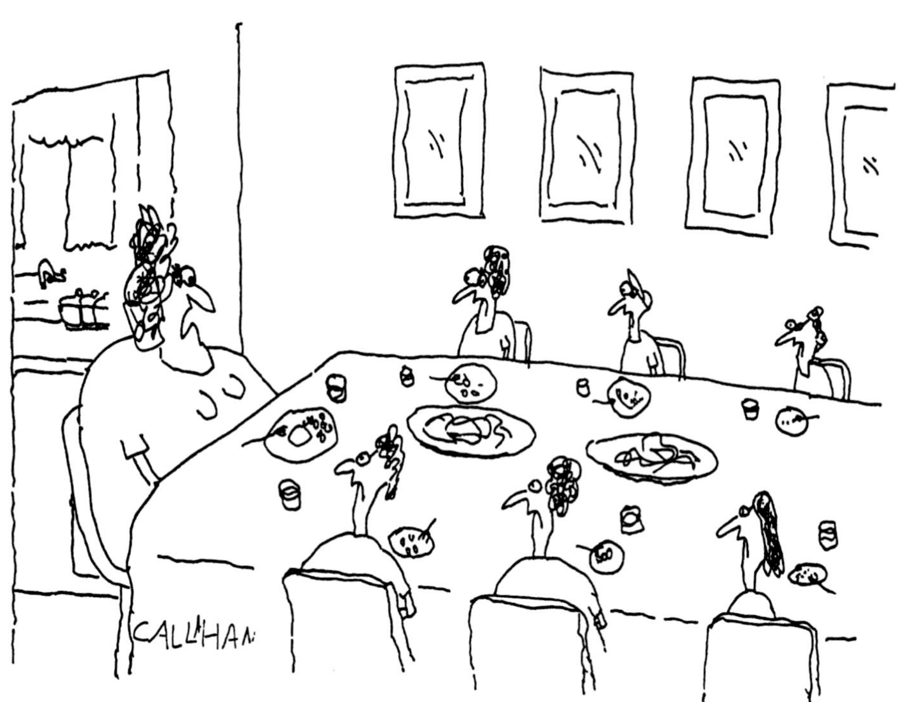

"Finish your vegetables! There are children in Beverly Hills with eating disorders."

HERMAN®

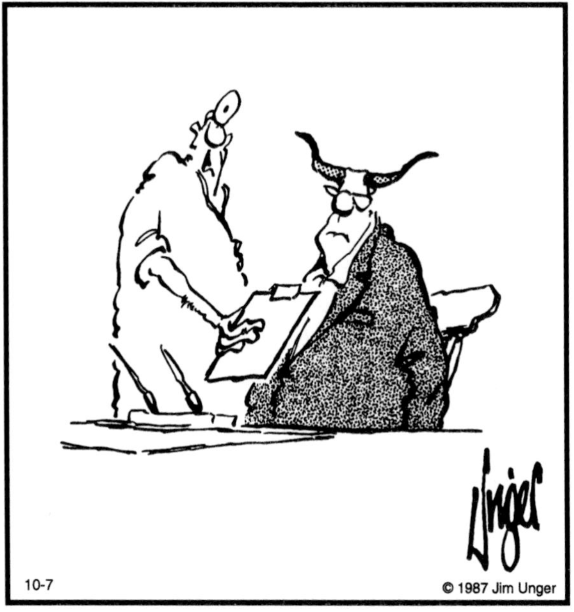

"You have to cut down on beef."

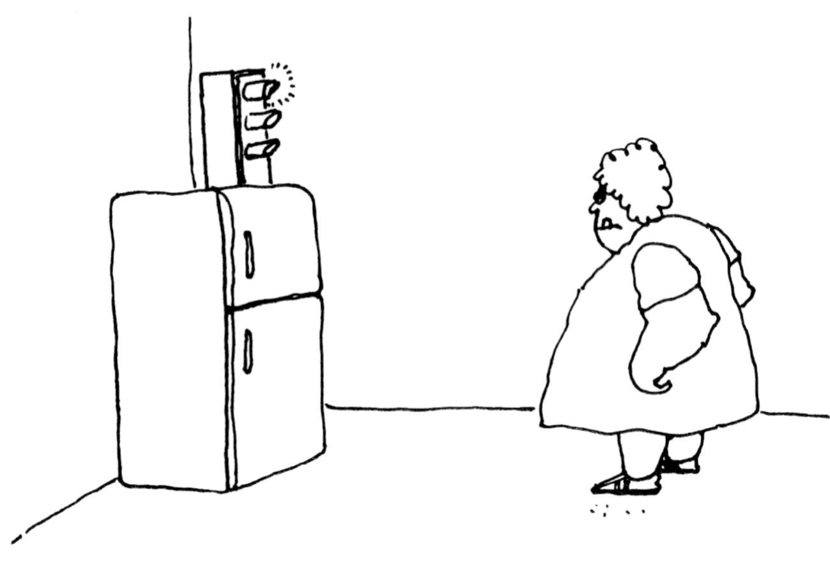

callahan

15.

Chronologically Gifted

Old, but not forgotten

Growing old

Geriatric encounters

FZZZT!
2-27
© 1996 John McPherson/Dist. by Universal Press Syndicate
McPHERSON

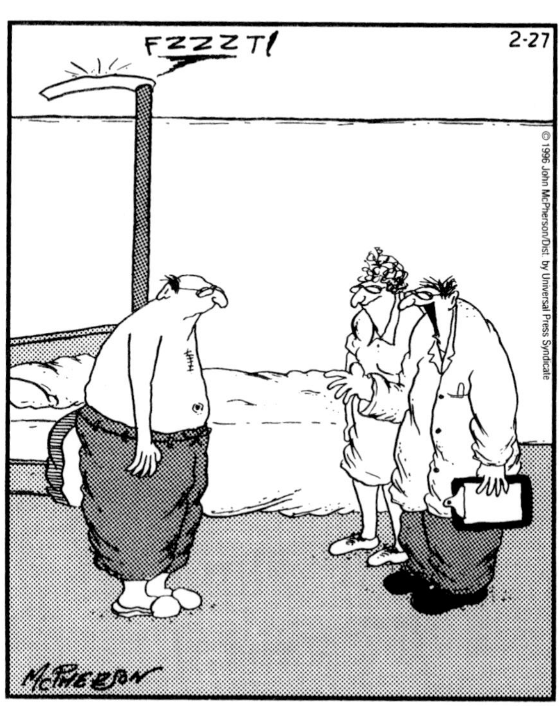

"Your new pacemaker operates on the same principle as a bumper car at an amusement park."

I'M GLAD TO SAY I'VE NEVER BEEN INFLUENCED BY THE VIOLENCE.
TOO BAD, THOUGH, ABOUT THE SEX.
S. Harris

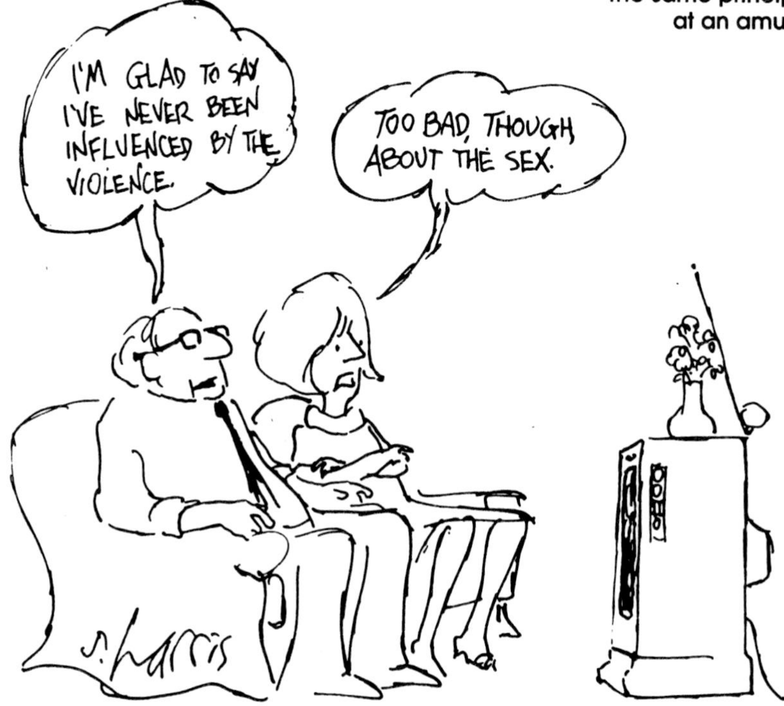

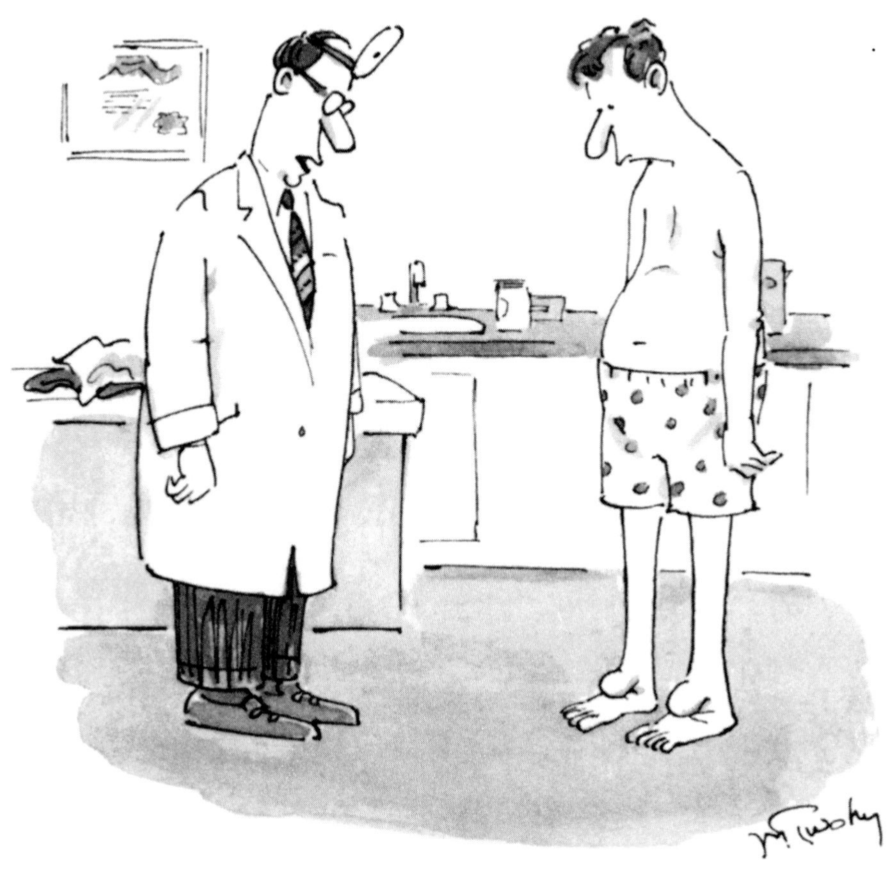

"The knees are the first thing to go."

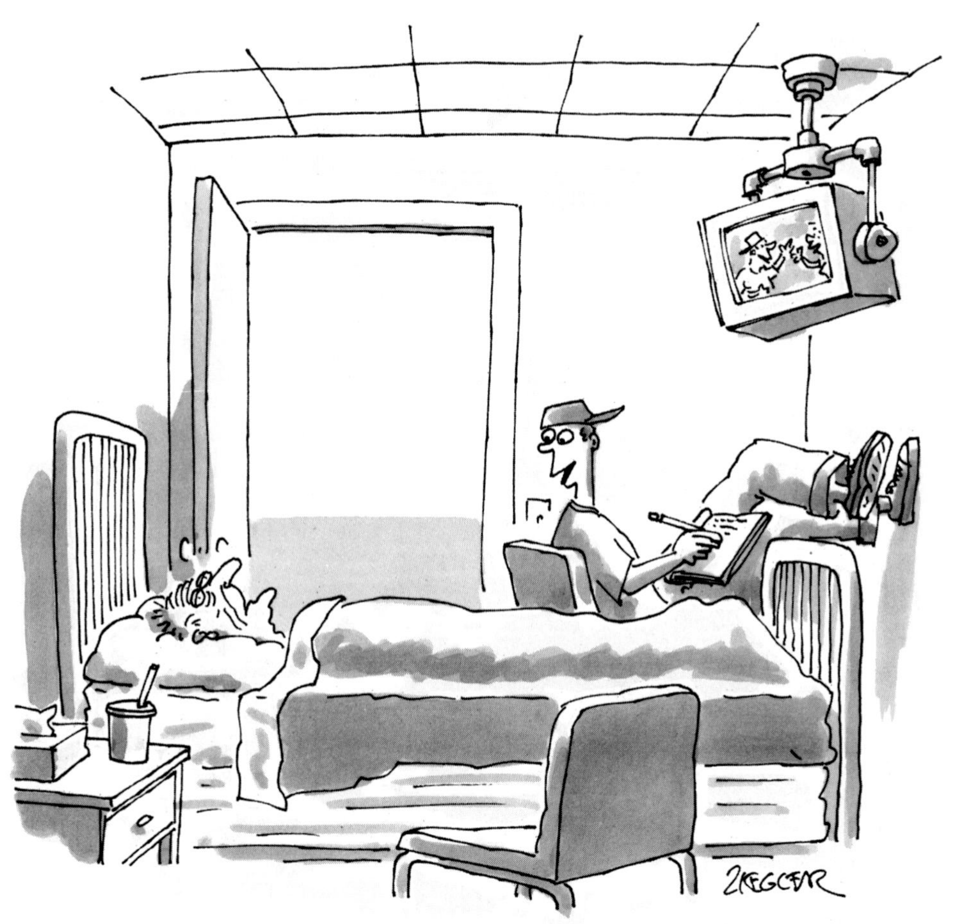

"Hey, Gramps, is 'deathbed' one word or two?"

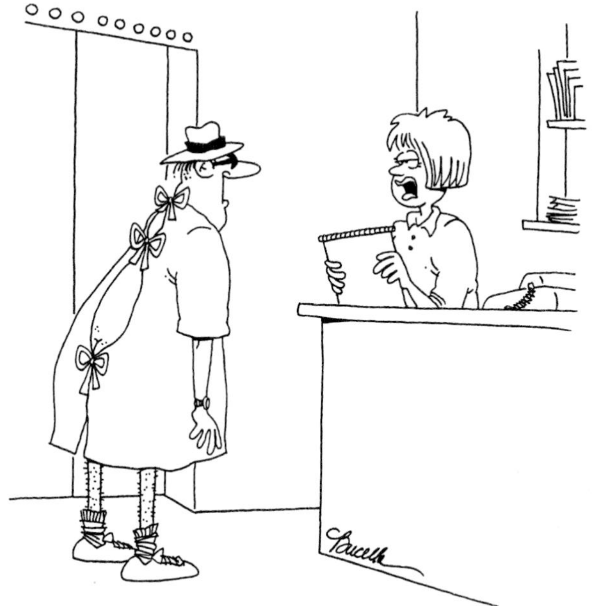

"I'm sorry, Mr. Nero, but visiting hours are for people who want to visit you."

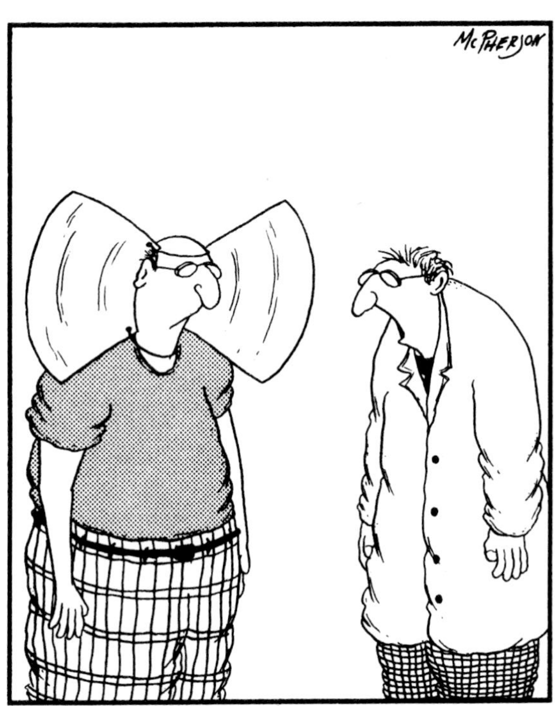

"Unfortunately, Mr. Mendrick, your insurance doesn't cover some of the more conventional hearing aids."

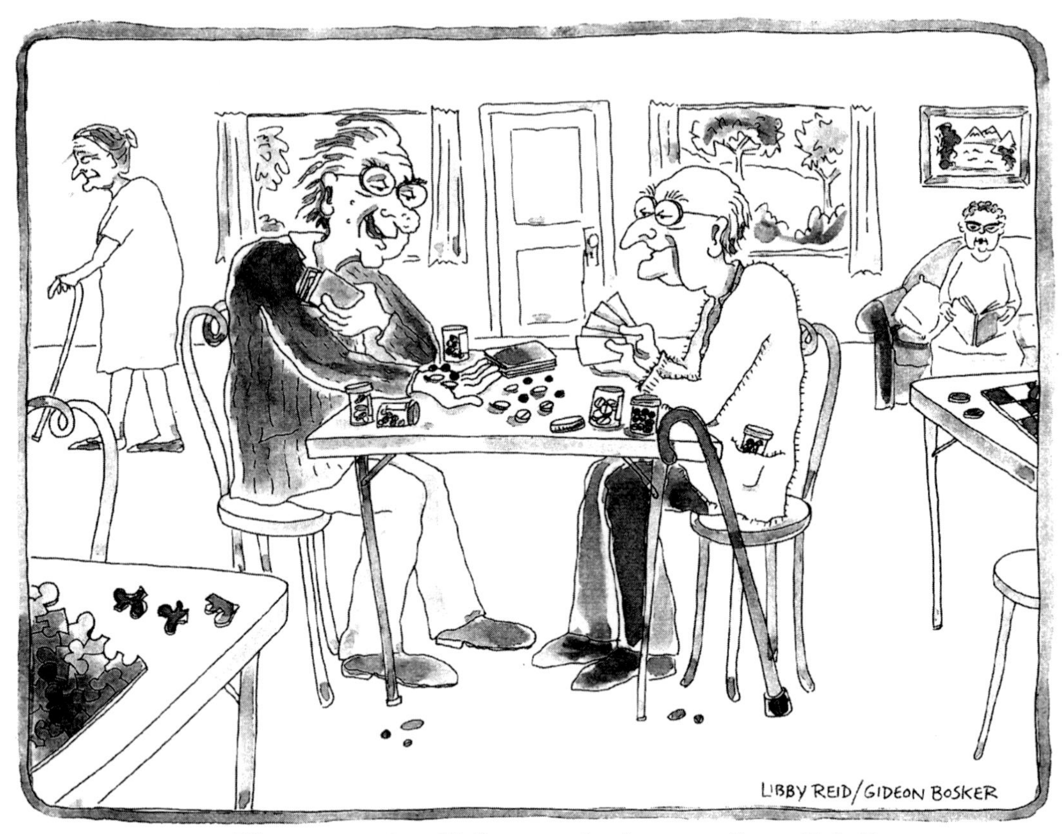

I'll see your two Valium, and raise you three Zoloft.

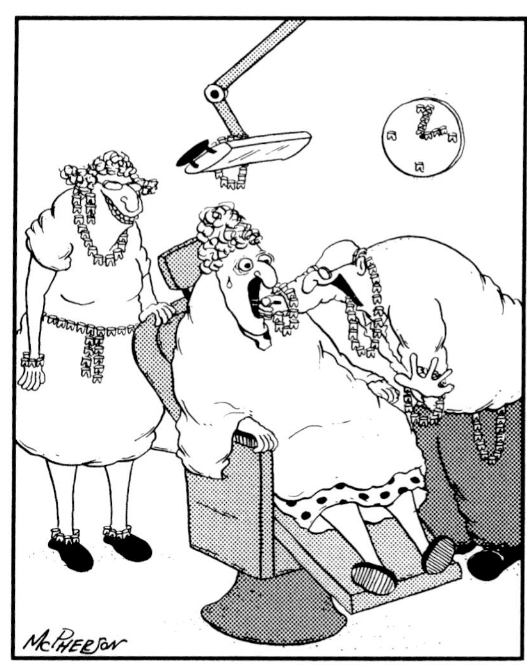

"Oh, my! This is *much* worse than I thought! I'm afraid we may have to pull *all* of these lower teeth! Take a look and see if you agree, Ms. Comstock."

HERMAN®

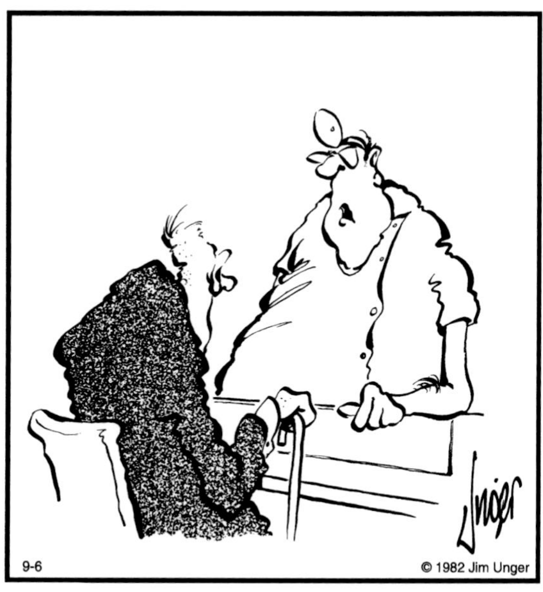

"Look, you're 103 years old, you've got to start taking better care of yourself."

IN THE BLEACHERS

By Steve Moore

© 1996 Universal Press Syndicate
www.uexpress.com
...WHEN I PLAYED FOOTBALL, WE DIDN'T WEAR HELMETS... WHEN I PLAYED FOOTBALL, WE DIDN'T WEAR HELMETS...WHEN I PLAYED FOOTBALL, WE...
12-20
JdSMOORE@AOL.COM
MOORE

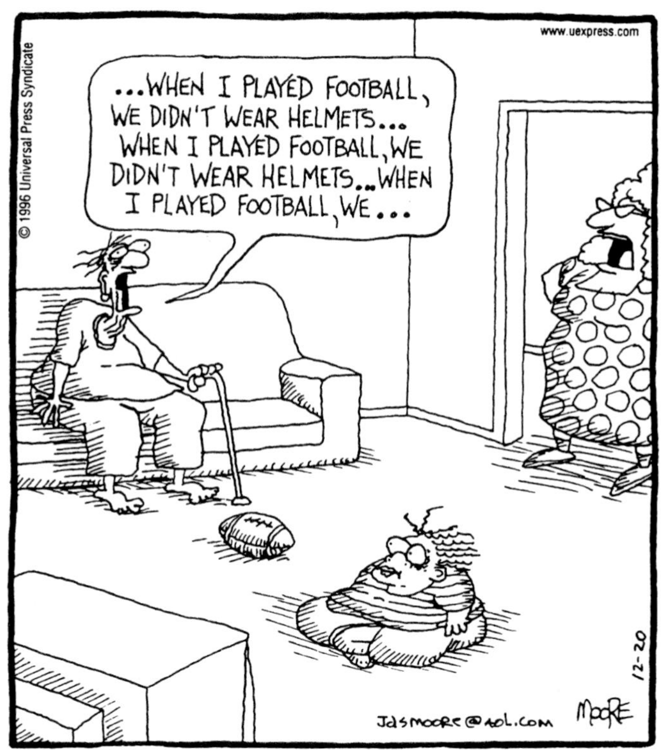

"Dewey! Grandpa's stuck again. Give him a couple of whacks upside the head."

16.

The Grin Reaper

Death and dying

Laughing at the funeral

Suicide made light

Humor in the morgue

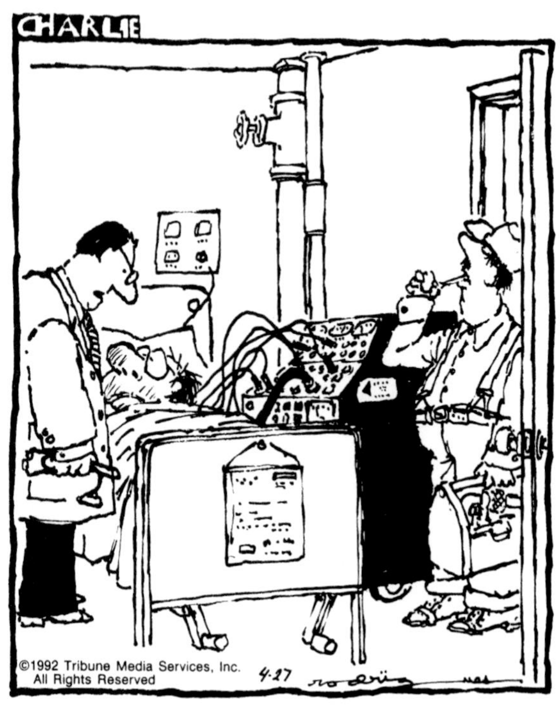

"Charlie, the plumber can't get to the steam pipes, so we're going to have to pull the plug on you."

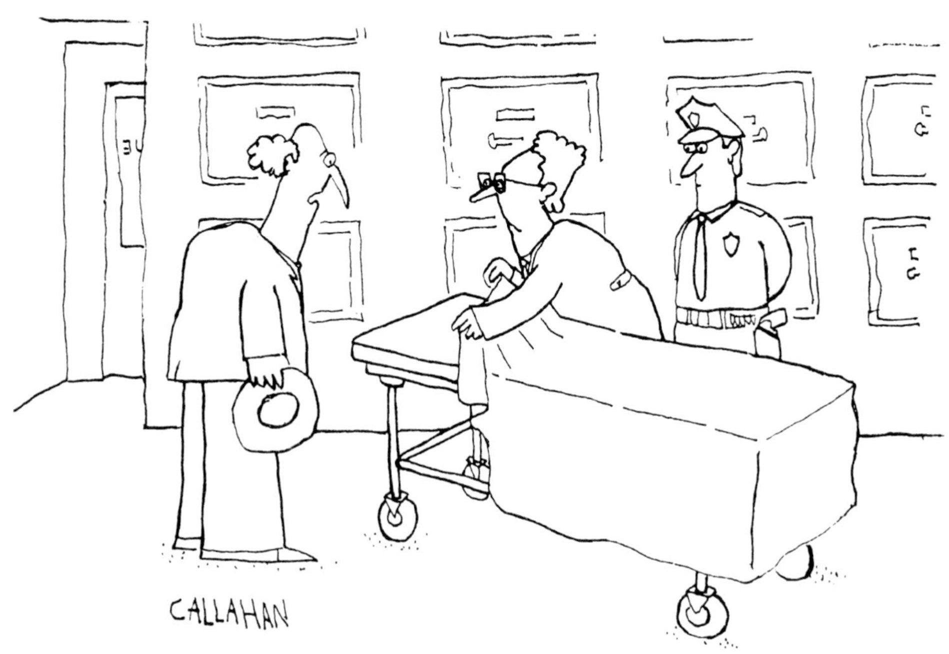

"Yes, that's my table."

IN THE BLEACHERS By Steve Moore

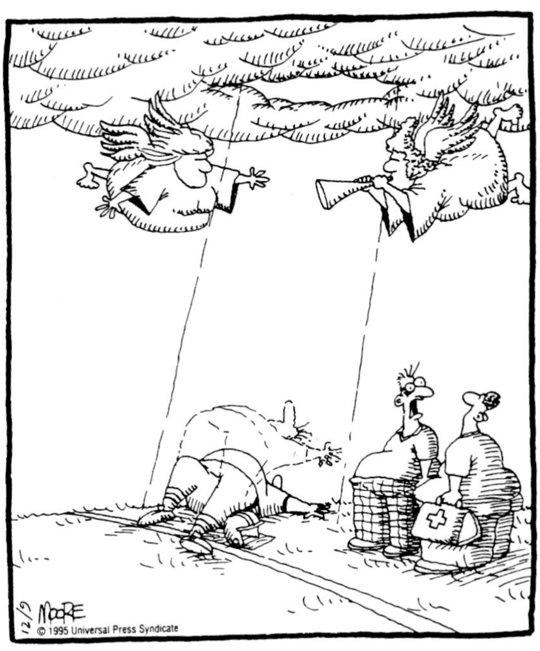

"Are you sure it's just a torn ligament?"

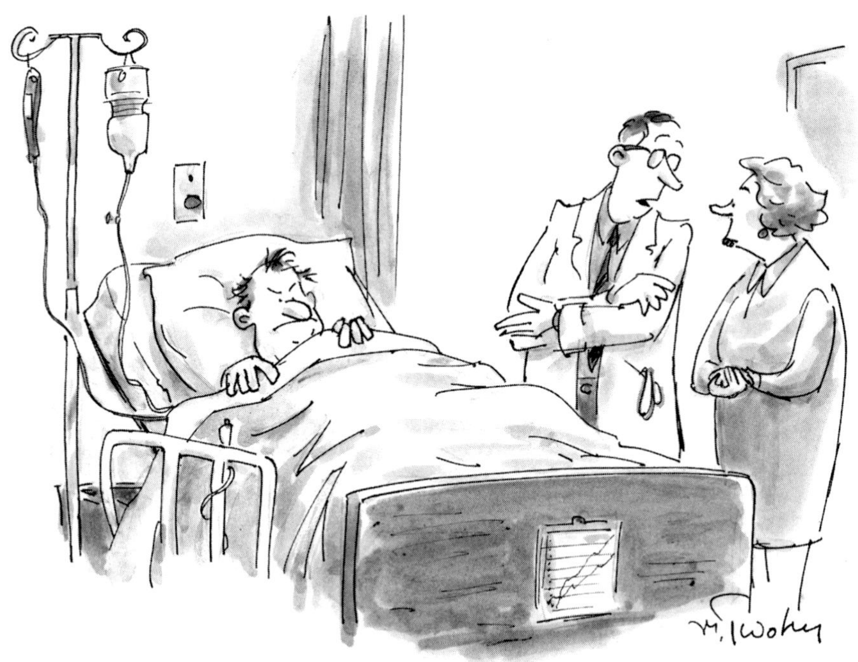

"He's one tough cookie. I've never seen anyone bounce back from an autopsy before."

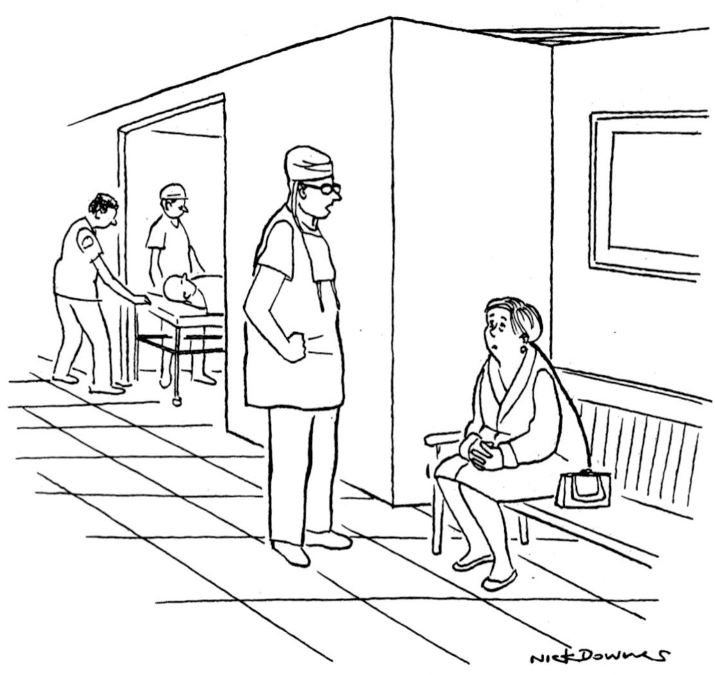

"I won't mince words, Mrs. Horton, concerning your husband, we've had a negative patient-care outcome."

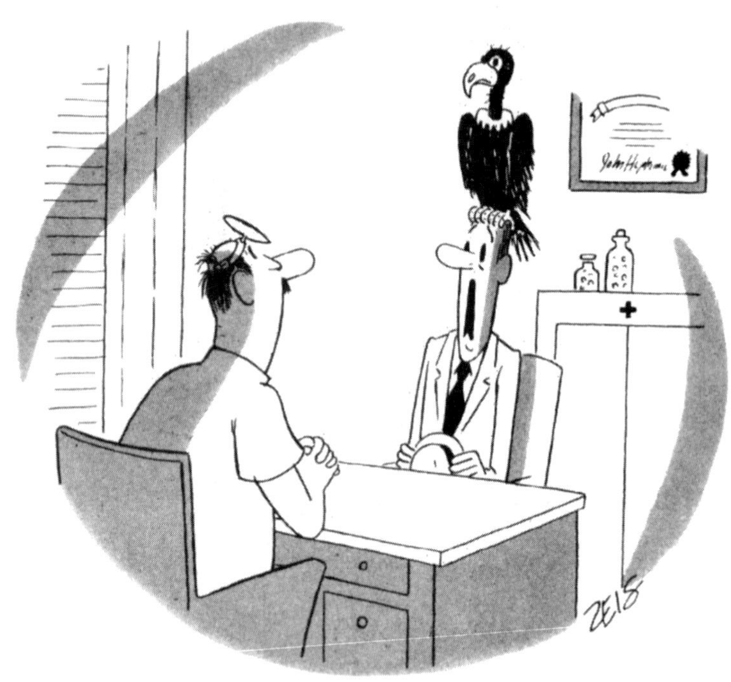

"I'm worried."

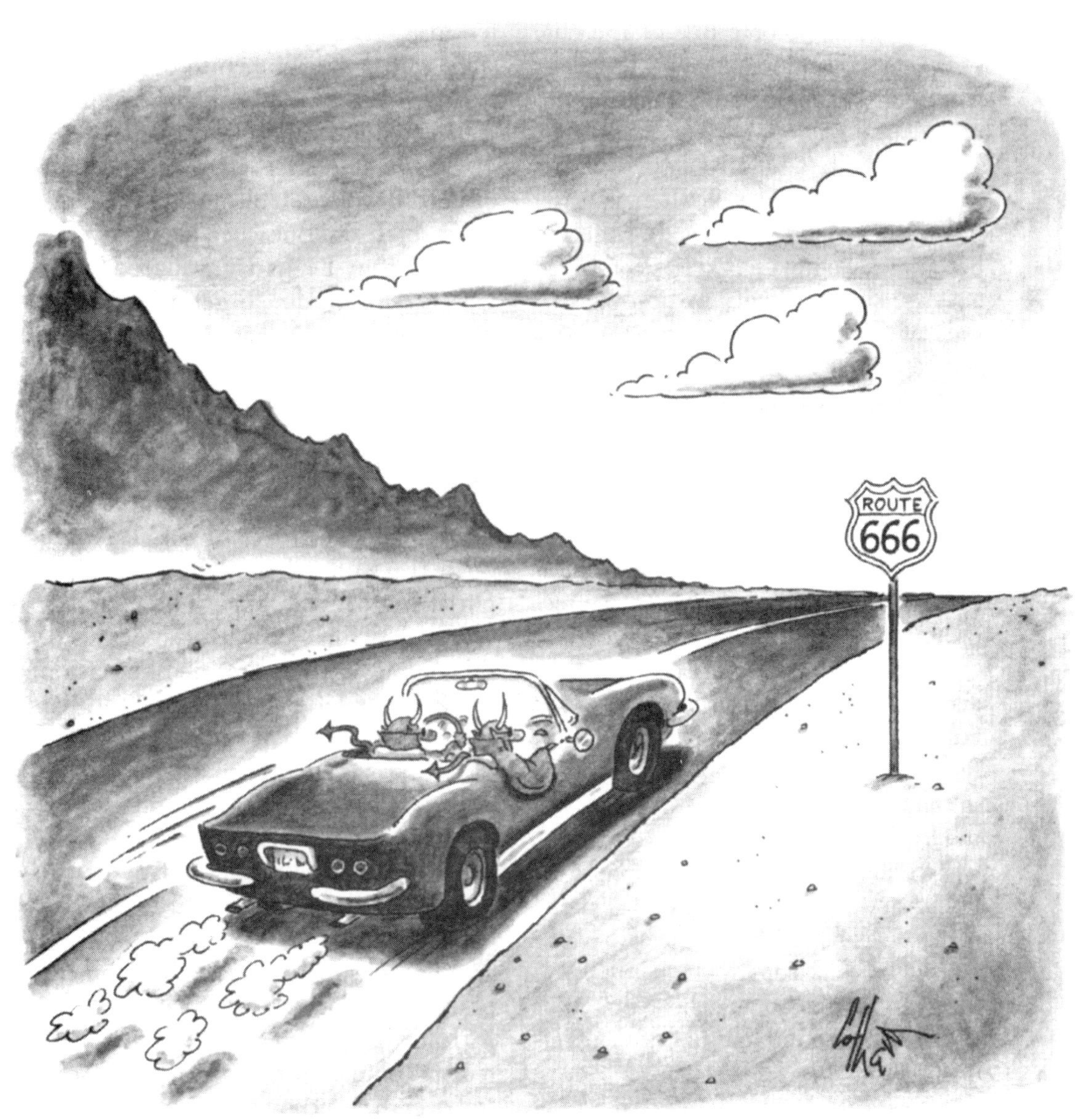
ROUTE
666

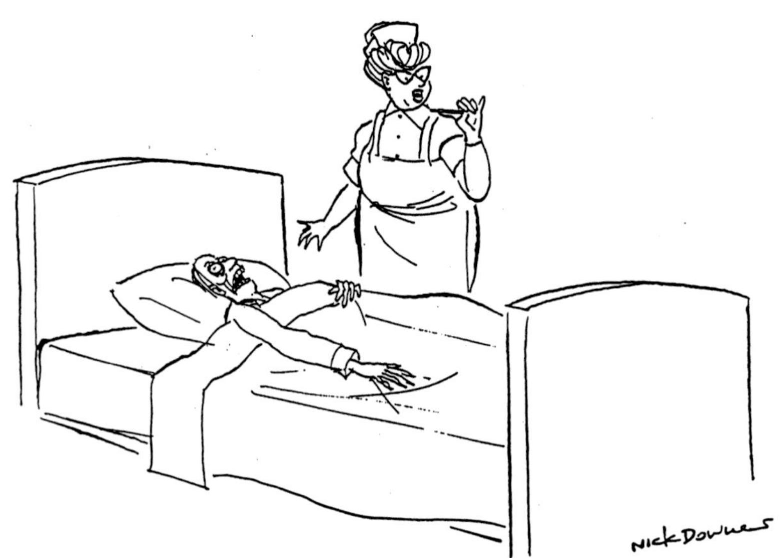

"Why, your fever's way down."

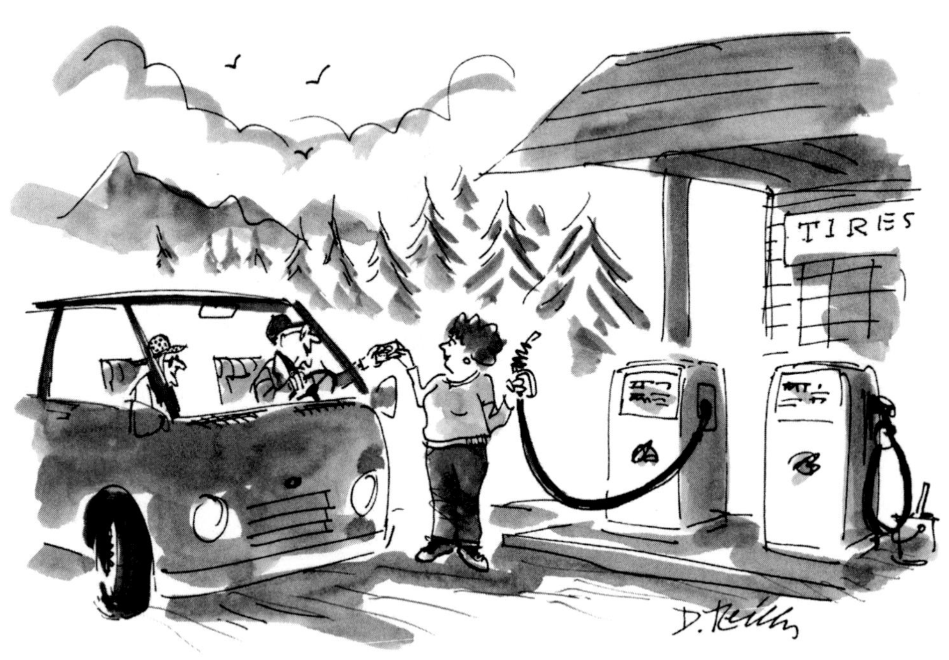

"Yes, Oregon's lovely, but we're just here for the suicide."

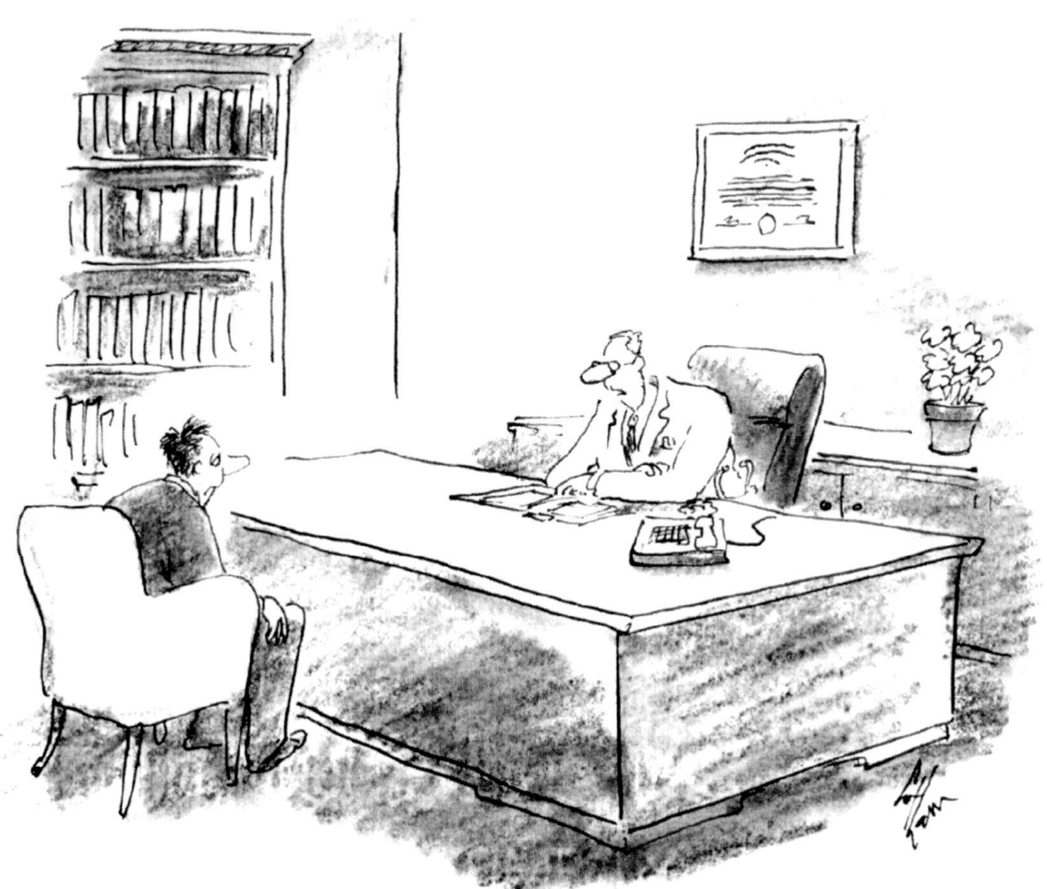

"I'm afraid the only procedure left open to us is embalming."

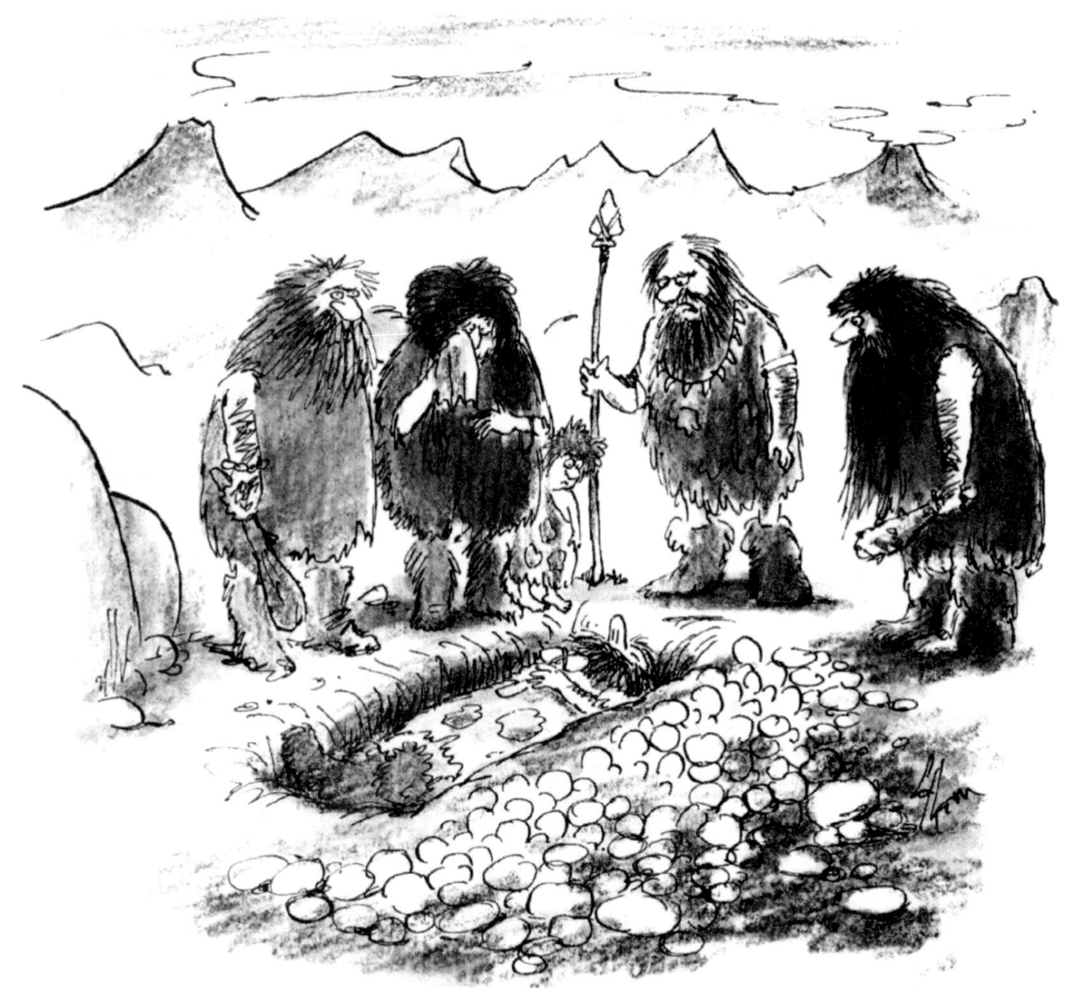

"We are comforted by the knowledge that at twenty-six years of age, he had lived a long and full life."

INCONTROVERTIBLE EVIDENCE OF REINCARNATION:
It's me-- Ted Layton from Sales... big guy, mean as hell, chewed you out a few times... had a heart attack 3 years ago...
SIPRESS

Nick Downes
"You're sure that's one of the stages of grief?"

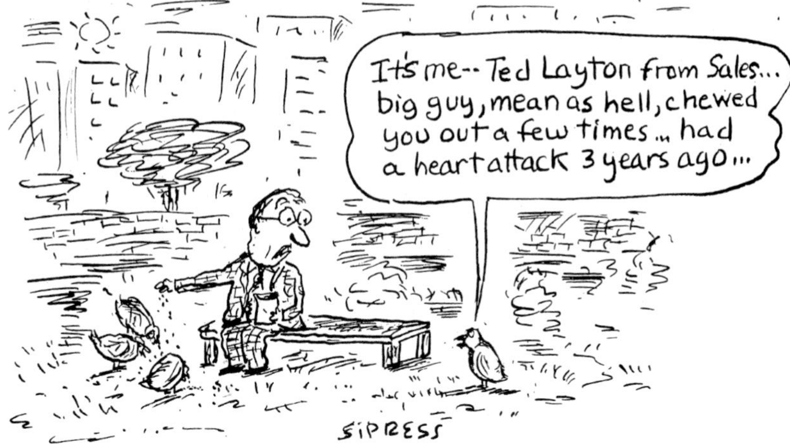

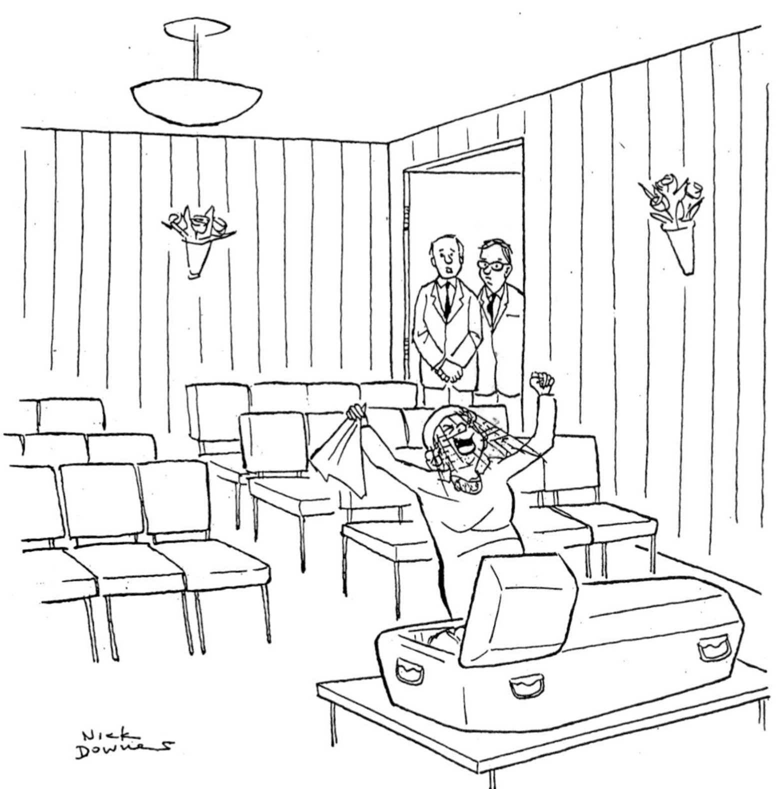

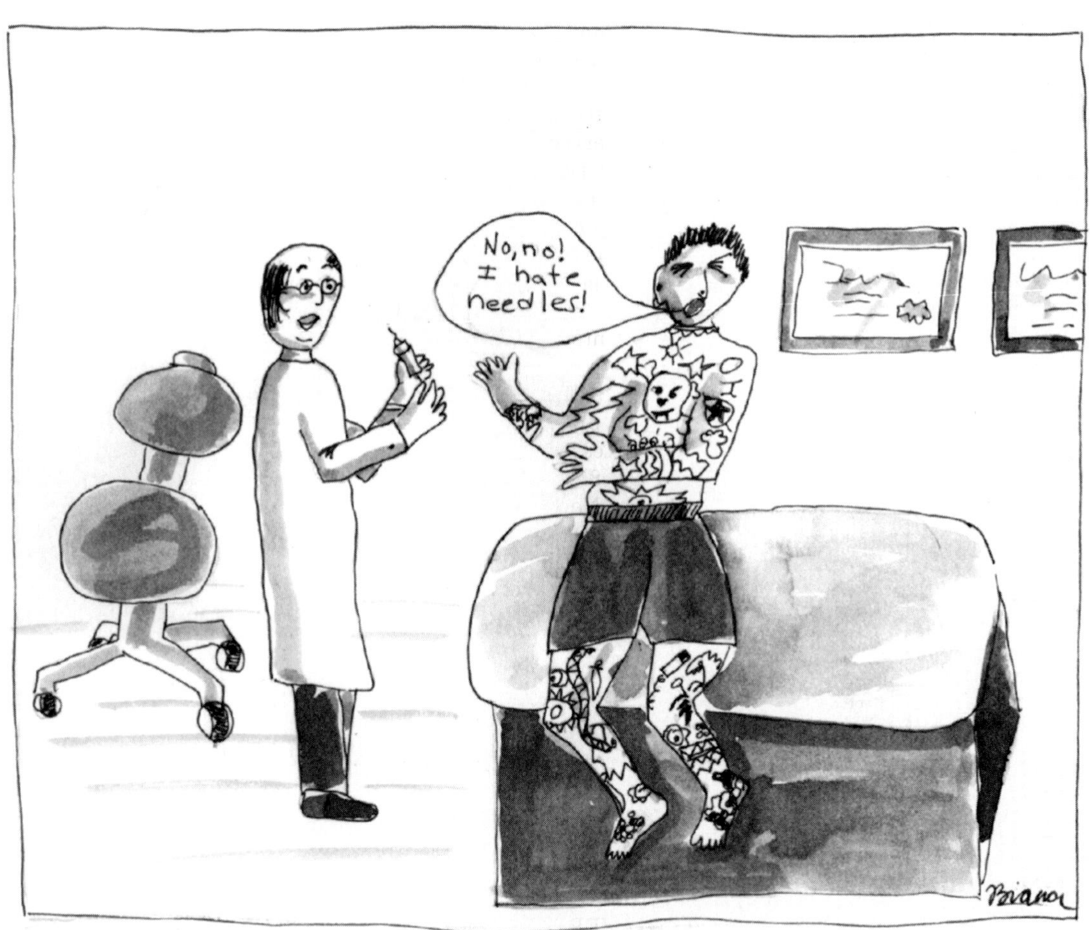
No, no!
I hate
needles!

CREDITS

Aaron Bacall p 82; Reprinted with permission from the artist, Staten Island, New York. abacall@msn.com.

Charles Barsotti pp. 41, 107; © 1997 from The New Yorker Collection. All rights reserved.

Brian Basset p 49. ADAM reprinted with permission of UNIVERSAL PRESS SYNDICATE. All rights reserved.

Jerry Bittle p 70. GEECH Reprinted with permission of UNIVERSAL PRESS SYNDICATE.. All rights reserved.

Martin Bucella pp 71, 169. Copyright 1998. Reprinted with permission of the artist.

John Callahan pp 23, 45, 52, 64, 71, 146, 163, 164, 174.; Reprinted with permission from the artist. Portland, Oregon.

Roz Chast p 111;© 1996 from The New Yorker Collection. All rights reserved.

Thomas Cheney p 31. Reprinted with permission of UNIVERSAL PRESS SYNDICATE. All rights reserved.

Judge Cohen pp 38, 52, 127. Reprinted with permission from the artist. Richmond, Virginia. All rights reserved.

Frank Cotham pp 21, 22, 43, 79, 91, 177 © 1994, 1996, 1998 from The New Yorker Collection. All rights reserved. pp 17, 84, 179, 180; reprinted with permission from the artist, Bartlett, Tennessee

Michael Crawford pp ix, 56;© 1994, 1998 from The New Yorker Collection. All rights reserved.

Eldon Dedini p 8;© 1997 from The New Yorker Collection. All rights reserved.

John Deering p 80; Reprinted with Arkansas Democrat-Gazette, Little Rock, Arkansas

Nick Downes pp 11, 23, 38, 39, 59, 62, 69, 72, 117, 127, 176, 178, 181. Reprinted with permission from the artist, Brooklyn, New York.

Benita Epstein pp viii, xii, 10, 18, 69. Reprinted with permission from artist. Cardiff-by-the-Sea, California.

Ted Goff pp 66, 74, 78, 154 Reprinted with permission of the artist, Kansas City, Missouri.

Steve Greenberg pp 67, 121 copyright 1993, 1996 Seattle Post Intelligencer

J. B Handelsman pp 105, 128;© 1997 from The New Yorker Collection. All rights reserved.

Sidney Harris pp 5, 9, 16, 18, 25, 26, 28, 30, 39, 46, 51, 109, 110, 158, 166. Reprinted with permission from the artist. New Haven, Connecticut.

Bill Harrison p 40; Reprinted with permission. Saturday Evening Post, Indianapolis, Indiana.

Gary Larson pp 34, 48, 65; THE FAR SIDE copyright 1990, 1994 FARWORKS, Inc. Distributed by UNIVERSAL PRESS SYNDICATE. Reprinted with permission. All rights reserved.

Bianca Lencek-Bosker p 182; Reprinted with permission from the artist. Portland, Oregon.

Robert Mankoff pp 36, 86, 138;© 1983, 1993, 1998 from The New Yorker Collection. All rights reserved. p 141 © 1998 from The Cartoon Bank, Hastings-Upon-Hudson, New York. All rights reserved.

Joe Martin pp 3, 148, 153; MISTER BOFFO. Distributed by UNIVERSAL PRESS SYNDICATE. Reprinted with permission. All rights reserved.

Michael Maslin p 2;© 1997 from The New Yorker Collection. All rights reserved.

Charles McLaren pp 28, 42, 68. Reprinted with permission from the artist. Bay Shore, New York

John McPherson pp 6, 12, 15, 20, 26, 29, 32, 48, 59, 62, 76, 82, 84, 87, 89, 90, 93, 94, 97, 99, 101, 102, 108, 110, 112, 114, 115, 117, 120, 122, 124, 125, 126, 130, 132, 133, 135, 139, 144, 147, 148, 150, 152, 155, 156, 166, 169, 171. CLOSE TO HOME copyright John McPherson. Reprinted with permission of UNIVERSAL PRESS SYNDICATE. All rights reserved.

C R E D I T S

Wiley Miller & Susan Dewar	pp 61, 159. US & THEM. Reprinted with permission of UNIVERSAL PRESS SYNDICATE. All rights reserved.
Steve Moore	pp 4, 27, 29, 37, 50, 134, 143, 151, 153, 172, 175. IN THE BLEACHERS. Reprinted with permission of UNIVERSAL PRESS SYNDICATE. All rights reserved.
Normal Dog	p 55.
Dan Piraro	pp 16, 37, 75, 108 BIZARRO. Reprinted with permission of UNIVERSAL PRESS SYNDICATE. All rights reserved.
Libby Reid & Gideon Bosker	pp 68, 111, 113, 14, 116, 170; Reprinted with permission from the artist, Portland, Oregon
Donald Reilly	p 178; © 1998 from The New Yorker Collection. All rights reserved.
J.P. Rini	pp 60, 160; © 1998, Reprinted with permissions from Cartoon Bank, Hastings-on-Hudson, New York. All rights reserved.
Charles Rodrigues	pp 9, 20, 25, 54, 90, 107, 122, 131, 159, 174; CHARLIE Reprinted with permission from the artist, Mattapoisett, Massachusetts.
Dan Schwartz	p 44; reprinted with permission from the artist
Danny Shanahan	pp vii, 53, 78, 81, 83; © 1993, 1995, 1996 from The New Yorker Collection. All rights reserved.
Mike Shapiro	pp 118, 145. Reprinted with permission from the artist
David Sippress	pp xi, 34, 35, 36, 41, 42, 45, 46, 50, 61, 64, 81, 83, 104, 112, 116, 161, 181; Reprinted with permission from the artist, New York, New York.
Peter Steiner	p 24;© 1998 from The New Yorker Collection. All rights reserved.
Mick Stevens	pp 7, 14, 92;© 1997, 1998 from The New Yorker Collection. All rights reserved.
Stratton	p 120; Reprinted with permission from the artist.
Mike Twohy	pp 3, 74, 77, 167, 175;© 1993, 1995, 1996, 1997, 1998 from The New Yorker Collection. All rights reserved.
Jim Unger	pp 4, 6, 13, 30, 49, 57, 58, 70, 72, 77, 86, 88, 92, 96, 98, 100, 106, 123, 132, 133, 138, 142, 160, 164, 171. HERMAN Reprinted with permission from Laughing Stock Licensing, Ottawa, Canada.
Bradford Veley	p 66. Reprinted with permission from the artist. Marquette, Michigan.
P.C. Vey	pp 10, 15, 27, 31, 75, 87, 147, 162. Reprinted with permission from the artist, New York, New York.
David Waisglass & Gordon Coulthart	pp 35, 54, 80, 140, 150, 161. FARCUS Reprinted with permission from Laughing Stock Licensing., Inc., Ottawa, Canada
Dan Wasserman	p 123 Copyright, 1997, Boston Globe. Distributed by Los Angeles Times Syndicate.
Bill Watterson & Lance Aldrich	pp 13, 55. CALVIN & HOBBES. Reprinted with permission of UNIVERSAL PRESS SYNDICATE. All rights reserved.
Roy Williams	p 89; Reprinted with permission. Saturday Evening Post, Indianapolis, Indiana.
Gary Wise & Lance Aldrich	pp 94, 136. REAL LIFE ADVENTURES. Reprinted with permission of UNIVERSAL PRESS SYNDICATE. All rights reserved.
Jack Ziegler	pp x, 168; © 1998 from The New Yorker Collection. All rights reserved.